THIRD EDITION

CONGENITAL HEART DISEASE
A DEDUCTIVE APPROACH TO ITS DIAGNOSIS

D0104169

THIRD EDITION

Congenital Heart Disease
A Deductive Approach to Its Diagnosis

Burton W. Fink, M.D.
Past Director, Division of Pediatric Cardiology
Department of Pediatrics
Cedars-Sinai Medical Center
Clinical Professor of Pediatrics
University of California
Los Angeles, California

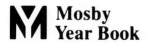
Mosby
Year Book

St. Louis   Baltimore   Boston   Chicago   London   Philadelphia   Sydney   Toronto

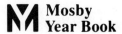

Mosby
Year Book

Dedicated to Publishing Excellence

Sponsoring Editor: Nancy Megley
Assistant Director, Manuscript Services: Frances M. Perveiler
Production Project Coordinator: Carol A. Reynolds
Proofroom Manager: Barbara Kelly

1   2   3   4   5   6   7   8   9   0   CLCDMA   95   94   93   92   91

Library of Congress Cataloging-in-Publication Data
Fink, Burton W., 1926-
    Congenital heart disease: a deductive approach to its diagnosis /
Burton W. Fink. — 3rd ed.
        p.   cm.
    Includes bibliographical references and index.
    ISBN 0-8151-3387-1
    1. Heart—Abnormalities—Diagnosis.   2. Pediatric cardiology.
I. Title
    [DNLM: 1. Heart Defects, Congenital—diagnosis.   WG 220 F499c]
RJ423.F56 1991
616.1'2043—dc20
DNLM/DLC   91-14167
for Library of Congress   CIP

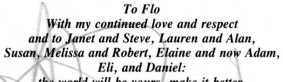

To Flo
With my continued love and respect
and to Janet and Steve, Lauren and Alan,
Susan, Melissa and Robert, Elaine and now Adam,
Eli, and Daniel:
the world will be yours, make it better.

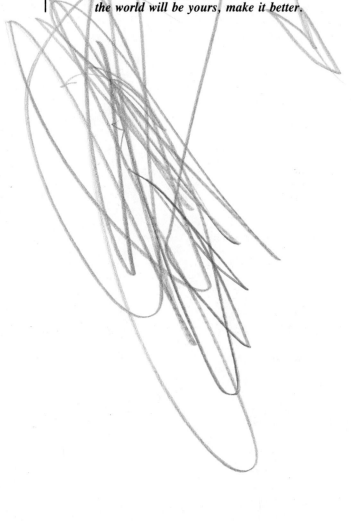

PREFACE TO THE THIRD EDITION

Since what I affectionately call "this little book" was first published in 1975, it has been translated into Spanish and Italian, and in 1985 was presented as an upgraded second edition. To have such continued acceptance of a personal effort over a 25-year period is indeed flattery of the highest order. After much personal deliberation and critical evaluation by unknown reviewers, the creation of this third edition seemed a reasonable and appropriate challenge.

Since echocardiography was introduced to the book with the second edition, the technique has been enhanced in a very powerful way by the addition of pulsed, continuous wave, and color flow Doppler interrogation. This has given the physician a noninvasive tool for the quantitative assessment of certain lesions that up to now have only been imaged. We must be reminded that echocardiography is basically an imaging tool. Each modality added to it must stand on its own when judged for value and usefulness. In my judgment, color flow plays a very real additive role in a selected number of lesions. In others, it likely could be defined merely as confirmatory or, when used inappropriately, confusing. In the light of these thoughts, examples of pulsed, continuous wave, and color Doppler images are selectively included in this edition.

One must immediately add that because of the enormous potential of echocardiography in the evaluation of congenital heart disease, the physician is at risk for using it to replace the basics of physical examination, electrocardiography, chest roentgenography, and most important, the thought process. That would be a mistake, indeed. The art of medicine incorporates all of the basics and adds to them new tools as they become available.

M-mode echocardiography has essentially been abandoned as a diagnostic tool, but remains useful for the inscription of images from which measurements of wall thickness, chamber size, and ventricular function can be elucidated. Therefore, reference to and examples of M-mode images have been left out of this edition.

Each chapter has been re-read and re-worked to make it as current and, at the same time, lasting as possible. For these reasons, the chapter on endocardial fibroelastosis has been eliminated. That entity having been diagnosed in the very early days of pediatric cardiology is now virtually never seen as an independent, presumably congenital entity, making its inclusion superfluous.

To increase the usefulness of the book, I have once again taken a personal liberty by inserting a chapter concerning the approach to a patient, generally an infant, with cyanotic heart disease. This short chapter and outline should help direct the physician to a specific later chapter for details.

This third edition, then, has continued to promulgate the basic principles expressed in the first and second editions and has added to it an update of present imaging techniques which will serve in their totality to increase the potential for accuracy in the diagnosis of patients with congenital heart disease.

I again wish to extend my enormous and never-ending gratitude to Norman H. Silverman, M.D., and A. Rebecca Snider, M.D., for their continued permission to use their original negatives of the two-dimensional echocardiograms reproduced in the text. All of the photographs and illustrations were once again created by members of the Department of Audiovisual Services at Cedars-Sinai Medical Center of Los Angeles. I thank them for their accuracy and diligence. I would also like to extend to Fernando Cano, CCPT, who executed the color Doppler work, and to Dolores Fisken, CMT, who tolerated my dictation in this edition, a very warm word of appreciation.

And lastly, though it may seem redundant, having been said before: to the medical students, physicians in training, practicing physicians, and allied medical personnel whose acceptance of the past editions has permitted the creation of this third edition, please accept my endless gratitude and a quiet and respectful thank you.

Burton W. Fink, M.D.

PREFACE TO THE FIRST EDITION

For the past 17 years I have had the privilege of teaching pediatric cardiology to medical students and house officers. I have long believed that the techniques that have been successfully employed in teaching by lecture and seminar would be equally effective in teaching by the printed word. This concept was the stimulus for this book. By designing the book primarily for the physician in training, I have taken certain liberties: it is short; each chapter is self-contained; treatment has been omitted; the language is less technical than it is literary; certain knowledge is presumed or not expected and certain data are idealized.

I believe if a person can envision the anatomic malformations that result from errors in embryologic development, a deductive approach to the diagnosis of congenital heart disease can be utilized. Thus, each chapter begins with the embryology and anatomy. A mnemonic then follows that links the anatomy and physiology in a diagrammatic line drawing from which the hemodynamics are developed and the clinical findings are evolved. The chapter ends with a differential diagnosis and a group of "pearls," which, by my definition, are items to which deduction cannot always logically be applied.

The book, therefore, in a very real sense, is as much one of method as it is one of facts. As such, it does not pretend to be either a definitive treatise or a reference volume. These types of texts are readily available and are listed in the bibliography.

It is hoped that because of the composition, size and teaching method employed, the physician in practice as well as the physician in training will find the book an easy reference for a brief review of an immediate problem.

Burton W. Fink, M.D.

CONTENTS

Preface to the Third Edition vii

Preface to the First Edition ix

PART I: LEFT-TO-RIGHT SHUNTS *1*

1 / Atrial Septal Defect *3*

Embryology *3*
Anatomy *4*
Hemodynamics *5*
Clinical Application *7*
Ostium Primum Defect *9*
Pearls *11*

2 / Ventricular Septal Defect *13*

Anatomy *14*
Hemodynamics *15*
Classic Ventricular Septal Defect *16*
Small Ventricular Septal Defect *20*
Supracristal Ventricular Septal Defect *22*
Eisenmenger's Complex *22*
Left Ventricle to Right Atrial Shunt *26*
Natural History of Ventricular Septal Defect *28*
Differential Diagnosis *29*
Pearls *30*

3 / Patent Ductus Arteriosus   *31*

Embryology   *31*
Anatomy   *31*
Hemodynamics   *32*
Differential Diagnosis   *38*
Pearls   *40*

4 / Endocardial Cushion Defect   *41*

Embryology   *41*
Anatomy   *43*
Hemodynamics   *44*
Clinical Application   *47*
Differential Diagnosis   *50*
Pearls   *50*

PART II: OBSTRUCTIVE LESIONS   *51*

**5 / Aortic Stenosis and Other Lesions Obstructive to Left
    Ventricular Outflow**   *53*

Embryology   *53*
Anatomy   *53*
Valvular Aortic Stenosis   *54*
Idiopathic Hypertrophic Subaortic Stenosis   *63*
Discrete Subvalvular Stenosis   *67*
Supravalvular Stenosis   *69*
Differential Diagnosis   *70*
Pearls   *70*

**6 / Pulmonary Stenosis and Other Lesions Obstructive to Right
    Ventricular Outflow**   *71*

Embryology   *71*
Anatomy   *72*
Hemodynamics   *73*
Clinical Application   *75*
Differential Diagnosis   *83*
Pearls   *83*

7 / Coarctation of the Aorta   *85*

Embryology   *85*
Anatomy   *85*
Preductal Coarctation of the Aorta   *86*
Postductal Coarctation of the Aorta   *91*
Differential Diagnosis   *97*
Pearls   *97*

PART III: RIGHT-TO-LEFT SHUNTS 99

8 / Differential Diagnosis of Cyanotic Heart Disease *101*
Pearls *105*

9 / Tetralogy of Fallot *107*
Embryology *107*
Anatomy *109*
Hemodynamics *111*
Clinical Application *113*
Differential Diagnosis *116*
Pearls *119*

10 / Tricuspid Atresia *120*
Embryology *120*
Anatomy *120*
Hemodynamics *122*
Clinical Application *124*
Differential Diagnosis *127*
Pearls *130*

11 / Transposition of the Great Arteries *131*
Embryology *131*
Anatomy *132*
Transposition of the Great Arteries With Intact Ventricular
Septum *133*
Transposition of the Great Arteries With Ventricular Septal
Defect *139*
Transposition of the Great Arteries With Ventricular Septal Defect and
Subpulmonic Stenosis *141*
Differential Diagnosis *143*
Pearls *144*

12 / Truncus Arteriosus *145*
Embryology *145*
Anatomy *145*
Hemodynamics *147*
Clinical Application *151*
Differential Diagnosis *155*
Pearls *157*

13 / Total Anomalous Pulmonary Venous Connection *158*
Embryology *158*
Anatomy *158*
Total Anomalous Pulmonary Venous Connection With
Obstruction *160*

Total Anomalous Pulmonary Venous Connection Without
Obstruction   *166*
Pearls   *171*

PART IV: MISCELLANEOUS DEFECTS   *173*

14 / Ebstein's Anomaly   *175*

Embryology   *175*
Anatomy   *176*
Hemodynamics   *178*
Clinical Application   *180*
Differential Diagnosis   *183*
Pearls   *184*

15 / Corrected Transposition of the Great Arteries   *185*

Embryology   *185*
Anatomy   *187*
Hemodynamics   *188*
Clinical Application   *191*
Differential Diagnosis   *191*
Pearls   *192*

16 / Hypoplastic Left-Heart Syndrome   *193*

Embryology   *193*
Anatomy   *195*
Hemodynamics   *196*
Clinical Application   *198*
Differential Diagnosis   *201*
Pearls   *202*

17 / Mitral Valve Prolapse   *203*

Embryology   *203*
Anatomy   *203*
Hemodynamics   *204*
Clinical Application   *206*
Differential Diagnosis   *212*
Pearls   *212*

Bibliography   *214*

Index   *217*

PART I

Left-to-Right Shunts

1

Atrial Septal Defect

EMBRYOLOGY

From approximately the fourth to the sixth week of gestation, the single atrial chamber is effectively divided into two. This is begun by the growth of a thin wall of tissue—the first septum—which originates in the dorsal wall of the single atrium and proceeds in its growth toward the endocardial cushions. These are concomitantly growing to separate the atria from the ventricles. As the first septum approaches these cushions, the space between the two structures is called the ostium primum, or first hole (Fig 1–1, A). As it proliferates to seal totally, fenestrations appear in the center of the first septum, leading to a second hole—the ostium secundum. At this time there appears a second thin septum growing to the right of the first—the septum secundum (Fig 1–1, B). The ultimate balance between proliferation and absorption in these two septa leads to the formation of a hole—the foramen ovale—to be guarded on its left side by a valve (Fig 1–1, C and D). This arrangement effectively permits blood flow from the right

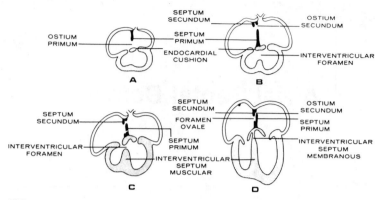

FIG 1−1.
Schematic representation of the formation of the interatrial septum. **A,** 30 days; **B,** 33 days; **C,** 37 days; **D,** newborn. (See text for explanation.) (Modified from Moss AJ, Adams FH [eds]: *Heart Disease in Infants, Children and Adolescents.* Baltimore, Williams & Wilkins Co, 1968, p 16.)

atrium to the left atrium during fetal development. After birth, when left atrial pressure exceeds right atrial pressure, flow in either direction is prevented.

ANATOMY

If there is an error in this development in either the amount of material laid down or the amount of material reabsorbed, a communication will result between the two atria, which is termed an atrial septal defect. If the interatrial communication is high in the septum near the junction of the superior vena cava and the right atrium, and if one of the right pulmonary veins drains anomalously into that site, it is entitled a sinus venosus defect. Should there be multiple fenestrations of the central portion of the septum, it is called a Chiari network. If the hole is in the center of the septum, it is known as an ostium secundum defect. If the communication is at the location of the ostium primum—the lower end of the septum—it is logically called an ostium primum defect. (The latter usually is accompanied by a defect in the mitral valve and can be classified as an incomplete atrioventricular canal or a partial endocardial cushion defect.) Figure 1−2 illustrates various types of atrial septal defects.

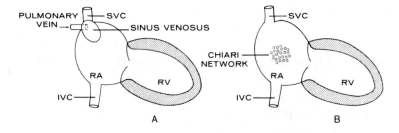

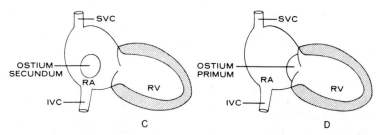

FIG 1-2.
Schematic representation of the various types of atrial septal defects. **A,** sinus venosus, **B,** Chiari network, **C,** ostium secundum, **D,** ostium primum. *SVC* = superior vena cava; *RA* = right atrium; *RV* = right ventricle; *IVC* = inferior vena cava.

HEMODYNAMICS

The patient with an atrial septal defect has a burden placed on the right side of the heart as a result of an increase in volume—enormous at times—coursing through the atrial septum from the left atrium to the right atrium. This is conceptualized in the mnemonic

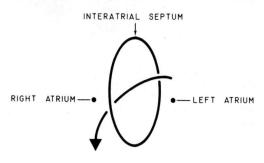

The arrow represents blood flowing from the left atrium through the interatrial septum into the right atrium. If the flow of blood is followed with the mnemonic in mind, the effect on the size of the various components of the heart can be demonstrated by the following diagram:

RIGHT ATRIUM ↑	LEFT ATRIUM →
RIGHT VENTRICLE ↑	LEFT VENTRICLE →
MAIN PULMONARY ARTERY ↑	AORTA → ↓
PULMONARY VESSELS ↑	

The arrows represent alteration in the size of a chamber or a vessel as follows:

→Unchanged
↑ Increased
↓ Decreased

This information can logically be translated to the chest roentgenogram, where one would predict an enlarged right atrium, right ventricle, main pulmonary artery, an increase in the vascular markings of the lungs, and a relatively normal left side. Such is the case as seen in

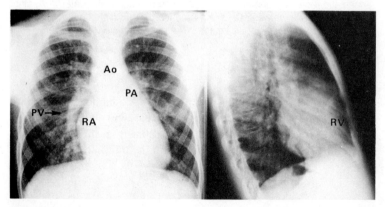

FIG 1–3.
Chest roentgenograms of a patient with an atrial septal defect. Note the cardiomegaly, enlargement of the right atrium, right ventricle, pulmonary artery and apparent decrease in the aorta. The pulmonary markings are increased. *RA* = right atrium; *RV* = right ventricle; *PA* = pulmonary artery; *Ao* = aorta; *PV* = pulmonary vessels.

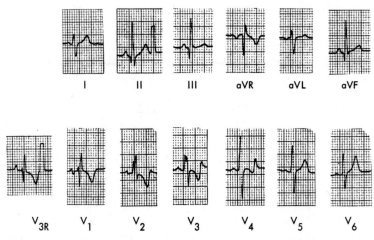

FIG 1-4.
Electrocardiogram of a patient with an ostium secundum type of atrial septal defect. The salient features are a dominant S_1 and RaVF, which is right axis deviation, and the rSR' in V_1 and prominent $SV_{5,6}$, which are interpretable as right ventricular hypertrophy. There are no Q waves in the precordial leads. (The right ventricular enlargement has caused clockwise rotation of the heart, displacing the ventricular septum well to the left.)

Figure 1-3. Although there are basic changes in volume, these are reflected in the electrocardiogram (ECG) as a form of mild right ventricular hypertrophy (Fig 1-4).

CLINICAL APPLICATION

The increased volume of blood presented to the right ventricle is ejected through the pulmonary valve in ventricular systole. This creates the typical ejection murmur, usually grade II/VI in intensity, which can be heard at the second left interspace and transmits along the course of the pulmonary vessels. This same volume of blood had passed through the tricuspid valve during atrial systole (ventricular diastole), leading to the frequently heard mid-diastolic filling sound in the area of the fourth or fifth interspace to the left of the sternum. The fixed overload of the right ventricle results in a prolonged ejection time of that chamber and consistently delays the closure of the pulmonary valve. This results in a wide splitting of the second sound. With expiration, venous return normally is decreased, but because of the fixed volume overload of the shunt, right ventricular ejection is not altered significantly. Thus, the second sound will retain its fixed splitting, being unaffected by respiration.

The patient with this lesion characteristically is asymptomatic. The appearance of the murmur will draw attention to its presence. The diagnosis can clinically be suspected in such a patient who may be slightly smaller in structure, is functioning normally, and whose chest is prominent on the left side, and who has an ejection systolic murmur at the second left interspace, a fixed widely split second sound, and perhaps a diastolic filling sound at the lower left sternal border. Suspicion would be intensified if the chest roentgenogram were abnormal as described and the ECG showed right ventricular hypertrophy. The expected enlargement of the right atrium and right ventricle can be demonstrated on a two-dimensional echocardiogram. The volume overload

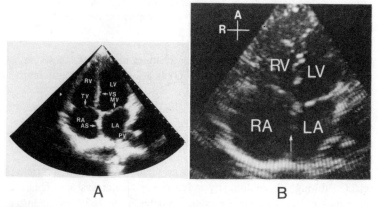

A   B

FIG 1–5.
Apical four-chamber view of an echocardiogram in a normal patient **(A)** and in a patient with secundum atrial septal defect **(B).** *Arrows* point to echo-free space in atrial septum. *A* = anterior; *R* = right; *RV* = right ventricle; *TV* = tricuspid valve; *RA* = right atrium; *LA* = left atrium; *MV* = mitral valve; *LV* = left ventricle; *LPV* = left pulmonary vein; *MB* = moderator band. (From Silverman NH, Snider AR: *Two-Dimensional Echocardiogram in Congenital Heart Disease.* Norwalk, Conn, Appleton-Century-Crofts, 1982, p 68. Used by permission.)

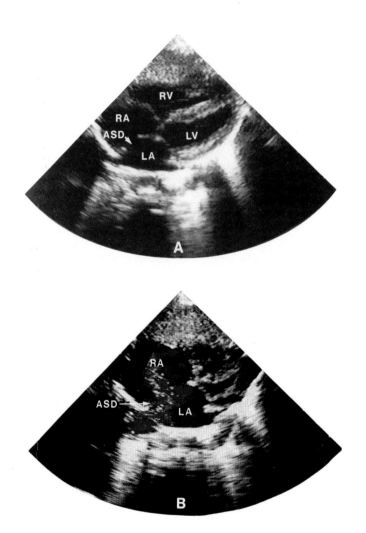

PLATE 1.
Subxiphoid view of an echocardiogram in a patient with an atrial septal defect **(A)** and a similar image with color flow **(B).** The shade of red represents flow toward the transducer, which is at the peak of the triangle, and shades of blue represent flow away from the transducer. Note the echo-free space in the atrial septum in **A** and the red color flow through a comparable space in **B.** *RA* = right atrium; *LA* = left atrium; *RV* = right ventricle; *LV* = left ventricle; *ASD* = atrial septal defect.

TABLE 1-1.

Idealized Cardiac Catheterization Data in a Child With an Atrial Septal Defect*

Site	Pressure (mm Hg)		Oxygen Saturation (%)	
	Normal	Patient	Normal	Patient
Superior vena cava			70	72
Inferior vena cava			74	76
Right atrium	a = 5 v = 3 m = 4	a = 5 v = 3 m = 4	72	85
Right ventricle	25/2	40/2	72	85
Main pulmonary artery	25/12	30/12	72	85
Systemic artery	120/80	120/80	97	97
Left atrium	a = 5 v = 7 m = 6	a = 4 v = 5 m = 4	97	97

*The salient features are an increase in oxygen saturation at the level of the right atrium, a slight increase in right ventricular pressures with a slight gradient across the pulmonary valve, and similar mean pressures in both the right and left atria.

in the right ventricle causes the ventricular septum to move paradoxically, whereby in systole the septum moves away from the left ventricular wall, and in diastole toward it—the opposite of the normal motion. In the subxiphoid or apical four-chamber view, the atrial septum can be visualized and the secundum defect imaged (Fig 1–5). Occasionally imaging of the atrial septal defect may be difficult, and the use of color flow will increase the ability to make an accurate diagnosis (Plate 1). Further confirmation of the diagnosis (when indicated) can be accomplished by cardiac catheterization during which an increase in oxygen saturation in the right atrium and equal pressures in the two atria would be found (Table 1–1).

OSTIUM PRIMUM DEFECT

The patient with an ostium primum type defect has all of the same physiologic challenges as one with an ostium secundum defect. In addition, because of the cleft in the mitral valve, mitral insufficiency is also present. This combination of events can cause poor growth and development and congestive heart failure in infancy. The diagnosis can be suspected in a patient who has all of the signs and symptoms of an atrial septal defect as discussed but who has left axis deviation in the ECG (Fig 1–6).

The subxiphoid view of the two-dimensional echocardiogram can demonstrate a dropout at the lower end of the atrial septum—the ostium primum (Fig 1–7). An apical view can also show the cleft in the mitral valve (not demonstrated). Results of cardiac catheterization will be similar to those of a patient with an ostium secundum defect. Because of the interplay on the lungs of the left-to-right shunt and the mitral insufficiency, higher pulmonary artery pressures may be present. The anatomical abnormality of the mitral valve and the degree of insufficiency can be visualized by angiocardiography.

Differential Diagnosis

The patient with an atrial septal defect must be differentiated from one having moderate pulmonary stenosis or an innocent murmur.

The murmur of mild pulmonary stenosis is similar but usually somewhat harsher and has with it a variably split second sound and frequently a diminished pulmonary component of that sound. The vas-

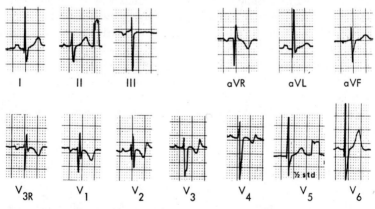

FIG 1–6.
Electrocardiogram of a patient with an ostium primum type of atrial septal defect. The salient features are a dominant R_1 and SaVF, which is left axis deviation, and the rSR′ in V_1 and prominent $SV_{5, 6}$, which are interpretable as right ventricular hypertrophy.

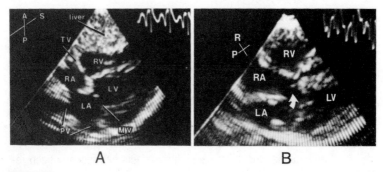

FIG 1–7.
Subxiphoid view of an echocardiogram in a normal patient **(A)** and in a patient
with an ostium primum atrial septal defect **(B).** (There is a slightly different orien-
tation of the two views.) Note the *white arrow* pointing to echo-free space in the
lower portion of the atrial septum between the two atria. In the normal subject
there is an apparent echo-free space in the atrial septum in the area of the foramen ovale. *S* = superior; *A* = anterior; *P* = posterior; *R* = right; *RA* = right
atrium; *TV* = tricuspid valve; *RV* = right ventricle; *LA* = left atrium; *MV* = mitral
valve; *LV* = left ventricle; *PV* = pulmonary veins. (From Silverman NH, Snider
AR: *Two-Dimensional Echocardiography in Congenital Heart Disease.* Norwalk,
Conn, Appleton-Century-Crofts, 1982, p 84. Used by permission.)

cular markings, as seen on the chest roentgenogram, should be normal. Cardiac catheterization may be necessary to differentiate the two.

The patient with an innocent murmur will also have a second
sound that is entirely normal. In addition, the murmur will vary considerably with changes in position and with exercise.

PEARLS

1. Atrial septal defect occurs more commonly in females than in
males.
2. The patients are, in the main, asymptomatic.
3. It is extraordinarily rare to have patients become symptomatic in
early infancy.
4. Patients with secundum atrial septal defect rarely go into heart
failure.
5. The development of marked pulmonary hypertension with rever-

sal of shunt flow is a late phenomenon and is very rare in the pediatric age range.

6. Right ventricular pressures in the catheterization laboratory in excess of 50 mm Hg strongly suggest a coexisting complicating lesion.

7. Because of rapid flow, mixing of the shunt may be demonstrated in the right ventricle rather than the right atrium. This could lead to an erroneous diagnosis of a ventricular septal defect. Clinical correlation is needed.

8. Atrial septal defect is seen commonly with the Holt-Oram syndrome.

9. Spontaneous closure of secundum defects has recently been reported.

10. Mitral valve prolapse may be seen in a substantial number of patients with an ostium secundum defect.

11. In a patient in whom the physical examination, roentgenogram, ECG, and echocardiogram all support the diagnosis of a secundum atrial septal defect, cardiac catheterization may not be necessary.

12. If the diagnosis of atrial septal defect is suspected and the ECG shows left axis deviation, an ostium primum defect must be seriously considered.

2

Ventricular Septal Defect

EMBRYOLOGY

Between the fourth and eighth weeks of gestation, the single ventricular chamber is effectively divided into two. This is accomplished by fusion of the membranous portion of the ventricular septum, the endocardial cushions, and the bulbus cordis (the proximal portion of the truncus arteriosus). The muscular portion of the ventricular septum grows cephalad as each ventricular chamber enlarges, eventually meeting with the right and left ridges of the bulbus cordis. The right ridge fuses with the tricuspid valve and the endocardial cushion, thus separating the pulmonary valve from the tricuspid valve. The left ridge fuses with a ridge of the interventricular septum, leaving the aortic ring in continuity with the mitral ring. The endocardial cushions are concomitantly developing and ultimately fuse with the bulbar ridges and the muscular portion of the septum. The final closure and separation of the two ventricles is made by the fibrous tissue of the membranous portion of the interventricular septum (Figs 2–1 and 2–2).

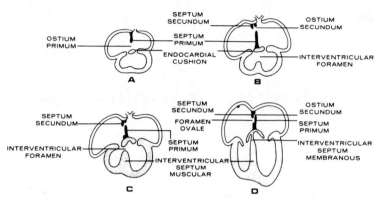

FIG 2–1.
Schematic representation of the formation of the interventricular septum. **A,** 30 days; **B,** 33 days; **C,** 37 days; **D,** newborn. (See text for explanation.) (Modified from Moss AJ, Adams FH [eds]: *Heart Disease in Infants, Children and Adolescents.* Baltimore, Williams & Wilkins Co, 1968, p 16.)

ANATOMY

Failure of adequate development of any of the component parts, namely, the muscular portion of the interventricular septum, the endocardial cushions or the bulbar ridges (truncoconal ridges), will result in a communication between the two ventricles—a ventricular septal defect. The defect between the two ventricles may lie above the crista

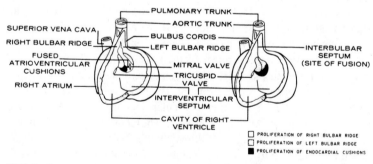

FIG 2–2.
Schematic representation of the role of the bulbus cordis in the formation of the interventricular septum. (See text for explanation.)

supraventricularis beneath the pulmonary valve, below the crista supraventricularis in the membranous septum, or below the crista supraventricularis in the muscular septum. The particular relationship between the membranous portion of the septum and the floor of the right atrium makes possible a direct communication between these two chambers. This permits an anatomical classification of ventricular septal defect into those above the crista supraventricularis, those below the crista supraventricularis, and those in direct communication between the left ventricle and the right atrium.

HEMODYNAMICS

Initially, the patient with a ventricular septal defect could be considered as merely having a communication between the left and the right ventricle, with shunt flow generally going from left to right. But a ventricular septal defect is not a simple lesion, because between the two ventricles sits the pulmonary vascular bed, which not only is influenced by the lesion itself but may exert its own independent influence on the lesion. To better understand this lesion, as well as patent ductus arteriosus and others, the various changes that take place in the pulmonary arterioles and their effect on pulmonary resistance need to be elaborated. Three different courses can be anticipated.

First, at the time of delivery and with the first breath, the lungs expand and the pulmonary arterioles dilate. There follows gradual resolution of the fetal musculature of the arterioles, with a drop in resistance occurring over several days to several months. The vessels finally reach their adult character, with a large lumen, thin intima, and reasonable musculature. These findings may remain unaltered despite the presence of a left-to-right shunt.

Second, after normal involution, the arterioles, in the presence of a persistent left-to-right shunt at the ventricular level, are the recipients of increased flow under an increased head of pressure, which may alter the pulmonary vessels by mechanical means, chemical means, or both. The vessels respond with hypertrophy of the muscular layer, followed by thickening of the intimal layer, which, individually or in combination, can cause elevation of the pulmonary resistance.

Third, in some patients, for reasons that as yet are not clear, the fetal vasculature fails to mature and the high initial pulmonary resistance remains elevated independent of any cardiac defect.

The intertwining of the location and size of ventricular septal defects and pulmonary vascular resistance is such that it would be wise to consider each variation individually.

CLASSIC VENTRICULAR SEPTAL DEFECT

Hemodynamics

This defect can be conceptualized in the mnemonic

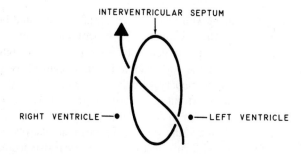

The arrow represents blood flowing from the left ventricle through the interventricular septum into the right ventricle and out the pulmonary artery. If the flow of blood is followed with the mnemonic in mind, the effect on the various chambers and vessels of the heart can be demonstrated by the following diagram:

RIGHT ATRIUM →   LEFT ATRIUM ↑
RIGHT VENTRICLE→ ↑   LEFT VENTRICLE ↑
MAIN PULMONARY ARTERY ↑   AORTA→
PULMONARY VESSELS ↑

The arrows represent alteration in the size of a chamber or a vessel as follows:

→Unchanged
↑ Increased

Translated to the chest roentgenogram, enlargement of the right ventricle, definite enlargement of the main pulmonary artery, an increase in the pulmonary vessels, and enlargement of the left atrium and left ventricle would be possible (Fig 2–3). The electrocardiogram (ECG) will vary from left ventricular hypertrophy (not shown) to combined ventricular hypertrophy (Fig 2–4).

Clinical Application

With the onset of left ventricular contraction, blood flows immediately through the ventricular defect into the right ventricle, lasting throughout all of systole and giving rise to a holosystolic murmur. It is heard best at the fourth interspace to the left of the sternum and will have widespread transmission throughout most of the anterior chest and even into the area of the pulmonary artery. It may be heard in the back by direct transmission. The shunted blood returns to the left atrium and may create a murmur in diastole as it flows through the mitral valve. This would be heard at the apex. The systolic murmur

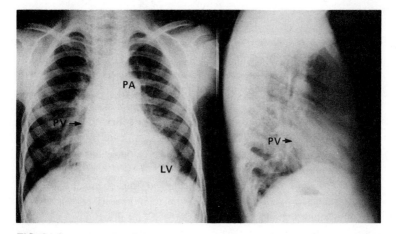

FIG 2–3.
Chest roentgenograms of a patient with a classic ventricular septal defect. Note the cardiomegaly, enlargement of the left ventricle, and the increase in the pulmonary artery. The left atrium is not clearly seen. The pulmonary markings are increased. *LV* = left ventricle; *PA* = pulmonary artery; *PV* = pulmonary vessels.

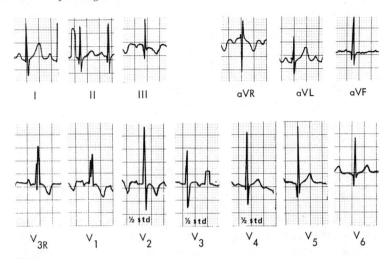

FIG 2–4.
Electrocardiogram of a 1-year-old patient with a classic ventricular septal defect. The salient features are a dominant R wave in V_1, a dominant R wave in $V_{5,6}$, and tall complexes in $V_{2,3,4}$, interpretable as combined ventricular hypertrophy.

usually is of such intensity (grade IV/VI) as to create a palpable thrill. The increased right-sided volume may delay closure of the pulmonary valves. Since the right ventricle will be influenced by venous return in addition to the shunt flow, the closure of the pulmonary valve will vary with respiration. The intensity of the closure of the pulmonary valves will vary directly with the degree of pulmonary hypertension present. The activity of the left ventricle will be reflected by a palpable thrust, felt laterally on the chest. If there is significant right ventricular enlargement, this will be demonstrated by a palpable heave to the left of the sternum.

An echocardiogram taken in the apical four-chamber view can demonstrate a dropout of echoes in the membranous portion of the septum beneath the aortic valve (Fig 2–5). Color flow Doppler has the ability to augment the image by demonstrating a shade of orange coursing through the defect from the left ventricle to the right ventricle (Plate 2).

Continuous wave Doppler is able to record the peak flow velocity

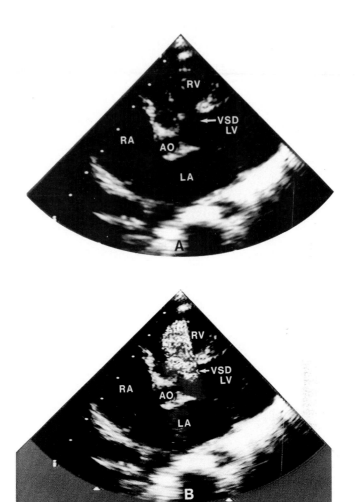

PLATE 2.
Subxiphoid view of an echocardiogram in a patient with a ventricular septal defect **(A)** and a similar image with color flow **(B).** Note the echo-free space in the ventricular septum in **A.** Note the red color and the mosaic pattern of yellow, blue, and orange coursing through the ventricular septal defect from the left ventricle to the right ventricle, that flow being toward the transducer at the peak of the triangle. *RA* = right atrium; *LA* = left atrium; *AO* = aorta; *LV* = left ventricle; RV = right ventricle; *VSD* = ventricular septal defect.

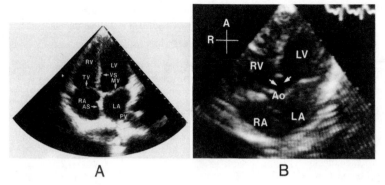

FIG 2-5.
Apical four-chamber view of echocardiogram in a normal patient **(A)** and in a patient with membranous ventricular septal defect **(B)**. Note the two *white arrows* pointing to the echo-free space in the high ventricular septum below the aorta. *A* = anterior; *R* = right; *RV* = right ventricle; *TV* = tricuspid valve; *RA* = right atrium; *LA* = left atrium; *MV* = mitral valve; *LV* = left ventricle; *Ao* = aorta; *MB* = moderator band; *RPV* = right pulmonary vein; *LPV* = left pulmonary vein. (From Silverman NH, Snider AR: *Two-Dimensional Echocardiography in Congenital Heart Disease.* Norwalk, Conn, Appleton-Century-Crofts, 1982, p 75. Used by permission.)

across the defect expressed in meters per second. From that number, using the modified Bernoulli formula ($4 \times \text{velocity}^2$), a numerical gradient can be mathematically determined. Therefore, once the systemic blood pressure is known, the systolic portion of which would be the equivalent to systolic left ventricular pressure, an estimate of the right ventricular pressure can be made. For clarity's sake, an example would be worthwhile: If a 1-year-old patient with a ventricular septal defect had a systemic blood pressure of 90/60 and the continuous wave Doppler recorded 3 m/sec peak flow velocity, the gradient across the defect would be 36 mm Hg (4×3^2). Therefore, the drop in pressure from left ventricle to right ventricle would be 36 mm Hg, making the right ventricular systolic approximately 55 mm Hg.

Cardiac catheterization will demonstrate an increase in oxygen saturation at the level of the right ventricle and minimally elevated pressures in the right ventricle and main pulmonary artery (Table 2-1). When pressures in the right ventricle are less than those in the left ventricle, the term "restrictive ventricular septal defect" is used.

TABLE 2–1.

Idealized Cardiac Catheterization Data in a Child With a Classic Ventricular Septal Defect*

Site	Pressure (mm Hg)		Oxygen Saturation (%)	
	Normal	Patient	Normal	Patient
Superior vena cava			70	70
Inferior vena cava			74	74
Right atrium	a = 5 v = 3 m = 4	a = 5 v = 3 m = 4	72	72
Right ventricle	25/2	40/4	72	85
Main pulmonary artery	25/12	40/14	72	85
Left atrium	a = 5 v = 7 m = 6	a = 5 v = 7 m = 6	97	97
Systemic artery	120/80	120/80	97	97

*The salient features are an increase in oxygen saturation at the level of the right ventricle and slightly elevated pressures in the right ventricle and the main pulmonary artery.

When both pressures are equal, the term "nonrestrictive ventricular septal defect" applies.

SMALL VENTRICULAR SEPTAL DEFECT

Hemodynamics

The mnemonic shown previously is applicable to this physiologic state as well. However, because of a small shunt and diminished blood flow, the effect on the chambers of the heart will be negligible and can be represented in the following diagram:

RIGHT ATRIUM→   LEFT ATRIUM→
RIGHT VENTRICLE→   LEFT VENTRICLE→
PULMONARY ARTERY→   AORTA→
LUNGS→

Since the alterations in chamber and vessels are negligible, it is predictable that both the chest roentgenogram and the ECG would be normal. This is indeed the case, and they are not demonstrated.

Clinical Application

One variety of this size of defect is Roger's ventricular septal defect. The classic holosystolic murmur located at the fourth interspace to the left of the sternum accompanied by a palpable thrill and a normal second sound would be expected. It must be emphasized, however, that other very small ventricular septal defects have their own clinical profile. In these, the flow through the defect occurs with the onset of systole but stops in the middle of systole, when muscular contraction of the septum may occlude the hole. This would give rise to a much softer (grade II/VI) early to midsystolic murmur localized to the fourth and fifth left interspace without significant transmission. The second sound would remain normal. At times, the murmur has a most unusual, literally puffy, sound to it.

If such a defect were in the muscular portion of the ventricular septum, an apical four-chamber view could demonstrate it (Fig 2–6).

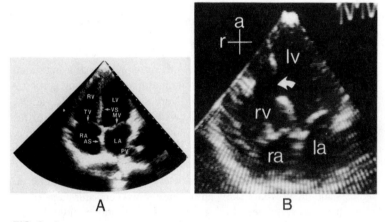

FIG 2–6.
Apical four-chamber view in a normal patient **(A)** and in a patient with muscular ventricular septal defect **(B)**. Note the *white arrow* pointing to the echo-free space in the septum between the left and right ventricles. A = anterior; R = right; *RV* = right ventricle; *TV* = tricuspid valve; *RA* = right atrium; *LV* = left ventricle; *MV* = mitral valve; *LA* = left atrium; *RPV* = right pulmonary vein; *LPV* = left pulmonary vein; *MB* = moderator band. (From Silverman NH, Snider AR: *Two-Dimensional Echocardiography in Congenital Heart Disease.* Norwalk, Conn, Appleton-Century-Crofts, 1982, p 78. Used by permission.)

Cardiac catheterization would show a very small increase in oxygen saturation at the level of the right ventricle. However, most patients in this group are diagnosed clinically and handled medically without catheterization.

Some muscular ventricular septal defects are not small and innocuous but rather large, creating hemodynamics quite like the classic membranous defect discussed earlier.

SUPRACRISTAL VENTRICULAR SEPTAL DEFECT

The peculiar location of this defect above the crista supraventricularis permits flow from the left ventricle almost directly into the pulmonary artery. Keeping in mind the location of such flow, one might expect that the murmur, also holosystolic in nature, would be higher in the chest at the first and second interspace to the left of the sternum, with transmission occasionally into the neck. This usually is not the case. The murmur, along with its thrill, most often is very much like that heard and felt in a classic defect.

The location of this defect frequently interferes with the support structure of the anulus of the aortic valve; this results in a high incidence of an early decrescendo diastolic murmur representing aortic insufficiency. The second sound would vary as that in a classic variety. The chest roentgenogram and ECG would be similar to those of the classic defect. The echocardiogram, however, can assist in the diagnosis and frequently will demonstrate the precise subpulmonic location of the defect. The presence of aortic insufficiency should direct one to this diagnosis promptly. Cardiac catheterization would clarify the diagnosis and likely would show an increase in oxygen saturations in the pulmonary artery or very high in the right ventricular outflow tract. Angiography, as part of the catheterization, would also have the ability to demonstrate the precise location of the left-to-right shunt.

EISENMENGER'S COMPLEX

By definition, this is a clinical situation wherein a patient with a ventricular septal defect (or any other left-to-right shunt for that matter) has developed sufficient pulmonary vascular disease and pulmonary hypertension to cause the shunt through the defect to become right to left.

Hemodynamics

The concept is demonstrated in the two mnemonics

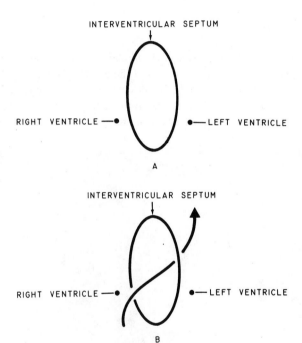

Remembering the definition of Eisenmenger's complex, the effect on the heart is demonstrated in A. When conditions worsen, mnemonic B applies. The effect on the chambers and vessels can be demonstrated in the following diagram:

RIGHT ATRIUM ↑   LEFT ATRIUM ↑ →
RIGHT VENTRICLE ↑   LEFT VENTRICLE → ↑
PULMONARY ARTERY ↑   AORTA → ↑
LUNGS ↑ ↓

Applied to the chest roentgenogram, one would expect to find an enlarged right atrium and right ventricle, an enlarged pulmonary artery, prominent proximal and small distal pulmonary vessels, and a left atrium and left ventricle varying in size (Fig 2–7). The ECG would demonstrate the dominant right ventricular hypertrophy (Fig 2–8).

Clinical Application

The generalized cardiomegaly will cause a prominence of the left side of the chest and a displacement of the apical impulse laterally and downward. Enlargement of the right ventricle will be recognized by a palpable heave along the left sternal border and enlargement of the left ventricle by a palpable thrust at the apex. The development of pulmo-

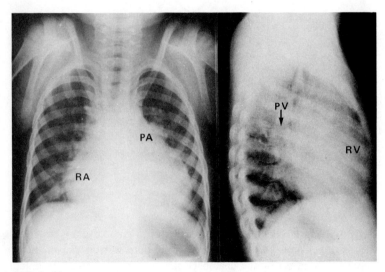

FIG 2–7.
Chest roentgenograms of a patient with Eisenmenger's complex. Note the gross cardiomegaly and increase in size of the right atrium, right ventricle, and pulmonary artery. The proximal pulmonary vessels are dilated, whereas the distal vessels are normal in size. *RA* = right atrium; *RV* = right ventricle; *PA* = pulmonary artery; *PV* = pulmonary vessels.

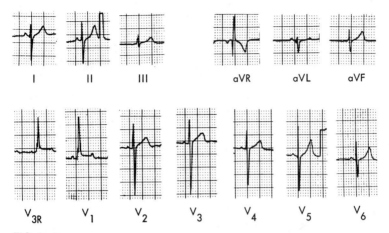

| I | II | III | | aVR | aVL | aVF |

| V_{3R} | V_1 | V_2 | V_3 | V_4 | V_5 | V_6 |

FIG 2–8.

Electrocardiogram of a patient with Eisenmenger's complex. The salient features are the dominant S_1 and R/S_{aVF}—right axis deviation. There also is a dominant R wave in V_1 and S wave in $V_{5, 6}$, which is interpretable as right ventricular hypertrophy. The T wave in V_1 is also upright.

nary hypertension has caused the right ventricular pressure to increase to the level of the systemic pressure. There being no gradient between the two ventricles, no shunting would take place, and therefore no murmur will be heard. As the shunting diminishes, right ventricular ejection time shortens, permitting the pulmonary valve to close sooner. As pulmonary hypertension increases, the intensity of the pulmonary valve closure will increase also. Therefore, with Eisenmenger's complex, one can anticipate a very narrowly split second sound, with significant increase in the intensity of the pulmonary component. With time and progression of the disease process, pulmonary resistance exceeds systemic resistance and the shunt through the ventricular septal defect reverses, resulting in systemic cyanosis. Cardiac catheterization will demonstrate peripheral arterial desaturation and right ventricular and pulmonary arterial pressures that equal systemic values (Table 2–2).

TABLE 2–2.

Idealized Cardiac Catheterization Data in a Child With an Eisenmenger Complex*

Site	Pressure (mm Hg) Normal	Pressure (mm Hg) Patient	Oxygen Saturation (%) Normal	Oxygen Saturation (%) Patient
Superior vena cava			70	62
Inferior vena cava			74	66
Right atrium	a = 5 v = 3 m = 4	a = 11 v = 7 m = 6	72	64
Right ventricle	25/2	120/4	72	64
Main pulmonary artery	25/12	120/80	72	64
Systemic artery	120/80	120/80	97	92–82†
Left atrium	a = 5 v = 7 m = 6	a = 8 v = 10 m = 7	97	97

*The salient features are generalized decreased oxygen saturations in the right side of the heart with no increase at the level of the right ventricle. The systemic artery has a slightly decreased oxygen saturation at rest and a significantly decreased value† when stressed. In addition, the pressures in the right ventricle and the pulmonary artery are systemic in height.

LEFT VENTRICLE TO RIGHT ATRIAL SHUNT

Hemodynamics

This very special variety of ventricular septal defect can be depicted in the mnemonic

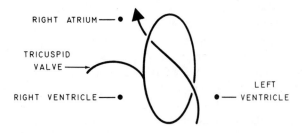

The arrow represents blood flowing from the left ventricle directly into the right atrium.

The effect of this blood flow can be shown in the following diagram:

RIGHT ATRIUM ↑	LEFT ATRIUM ↑
RIGHT VENTRICLE ↑	LEFT VENTRICLE ↑
PULMONARY ARTERY ↑	AORTA → ↑
LUNGS ↑	

Applied to the chest roentgenogram, one would expect to find an enlargement of the right atrium, right ventricle, pulmonary artery, and lung fields. The left atrium may be enlarged also, as would the left ventricle. The ECG would show combined ventricular hypertrophy and possibly right atrial hypertrophy and would resemble that seen in an atrial septal defect. These are not demonstrated.

Clinical Application

The similarity between this variety of ventricular septal defect and the ostium secundum type of atrial septal defect should be apparent. The chest might be more prominent on the left side, with a right ventricular heave, but a left ventricular thrust might be present also. The flow going from a high-pressure chamber to a low-pressure chamber would more likely resemble the holosystolic murmur of the classic ventricular septal defect. It would, however, be somewhat higher in the chest and would be accompanied by a thrill. The second sound would reflect the constant overload of the right ventricle and would more closely approximate that of the atrial septal defect. A wide split would be anticipated, and variability with respiration would be minimal.

The apical four-chamber view of the echocardiogram (see Fig 2–5, A) demonstrates the relationship of the tricuspid and mitral valves as they insert into the center, or crux, of the cardiac skeleton. The tricuspid valve is more apically oriented, which then places the floor of the right atrium in contact with the ventricular septum. Appropriate Doppler investigation and color flow can then demonstrate the shunt flow directly from the left ventricle to the right atrium, establishing the diagnosis (not demonstrated). Cardiac catheterization would be useful to define the lesion where one would expect an increase in oxygen saturation at the level of the right atrium. Left ventricular angiography would show the communication between that chamber and the right atrium.

NATURAL HISTORY OF VENTRICULAR
SEPTAL DEFECT

The information presented to this point now can be used to present an overall view of this anatomical entity and its variations, thereby giving a portrait of its natural history.

The newborn has virtually equal resistances in both the pulmonary and systemic circuits. The patient with a ventricular septal defect will be no different. His pressures in the right and left ventricles will be equal also, and no murmur can be expected to be present at birth. As the resistance in the lungs falls, there is a concomitant drop in the right ventricular pressure, creating a gradient between the two ventricles. The flow then can take place, and a murmur will be heard. The initial physiologic effect of the increased flow is to burden the left atrium and ventricle with an increased volume. If this occurs gradually, accommodation is possible and no clinical problem will result. If, however, the volume burden is acute and overwhelming, heart failure will ensue.

One patient may be born normally, have a murmur at 2 to 6 weeks of age, be totally asymptomatic, and grow in a normal fashion, keeping the defect but apparently unaffected by it. Another patient may be born normally, have a murmur at 2 to 6 weeks of age, be totally asymptomatic, and grow in a normal fashion, but by 1 year of age have the murmur disappear. This is believed to represent spontaneous closure of the ventricular septal defect and may occur in as high as 50% of patients. Another patient may be born normally, have a murmur at 2 to 6 weeks of age, and prove to have a clinically significant defect. With time, however, and through a mechanism not clearly understood, hypertrophy of the right ventricular infundibulum takes place. This patient will improve clinically, because the flow into the pulmonary circuit will be diminished. Another patient may be born normally, have a murmur at 2 to 6 weeks of age, and at that time or shortly thereafter go into heart failure. At catheterization, very large shunt flows will be present along with low pulmonary resistance (remember that resistance equals pressure divided by flow). These patients, when compensated, will grow but usually poorly. Some can be maintained to an age suitable for elective repair, whereas others will remain in such congestive failure that an early surgical approach will be required. A last group of patients will be born apparently normal, have a murmur at 2 to 6 weeks of age but grow poorly, although not necessarily suffer congestive heart failure. When catheterized, they will be found to have pulmonary resistances approaching systemic levels, with moderate to minimal left-to-right shunts. The troublesome fact is that it is impossible to predict which course an infant with a ventricular septal defect will take. Therefore, such a patient must be followed closely using all of the nuances of the physical examination, enlisting information gained from sequential echocardiograms, and, when necessary, resorting to cardiac catheterization to ascertain which course the patient is following.

DIFFERENTIAL DIAGNOSIS

The patient with a ventricular septal defect must be differentiated from a patient with idiopathic hypertrophic subaortic stenosis, a patent ductus arteriosus, an atrial septal defect, an innocent murmur, and noncyanotic tetralogy of Fallot.

The patient with idiopathic hypertrophic subaortic stenosis has a murmur that varies in intensity, occurs later in systole and is altered significantly by venous return, and is mentioned in the differential only because the location of the murmur is at the same general location as that of the ventricular septal defect.

The patient with an atrial septal defect is only momentarily confused with one having a left ventricle to right atrial type of ventricular septal defect. The absence of a thrill and the much quieter murmur should help make the differential. Cardiac catheterization should permit an accurate differentiation.

Although the innocent murmur of the "twangy string" variety is heard at the same general location, it is early, occurs in midsystole, and is lower in pitch and very variable in its characteristics. In addition, the patient will have a normal chest roentgenogram and ECG.

If the patient with a ventricular septal defect manifests secondary infundibular hypertrophy, he or she then will resemble the patient with noncyanotic tetralogy of Fallot. If the patient has been followed clinically, the appearance of a decreased pulmonary component of the second sound in the presence of right ventricular hypertrophy on the ECG will suggest the presence of acquired infundibular stenosis. If, however, such a clinical course is not known, a differentiation may not be possible.

In infancy, the patient with a patent ductus arteriosus generally has only a systolic murmur that may be indistinguishable from that heard in a patient with a ventricular septal defect. Echocardiography will help clarify the problem. Occasionally cardiac catheterization is necessary.

PEARLS

1. Ventricular septal defect occurs more commonly in males than in females.
2. The murmurs heard in early infancy, which disappear by 1 year of age, probably represent defects that have closed spontaneously.
3. Some patients maintain elevated pulmonary resistances despite therapy directed at the ventricular septal defect and may, in fact, represent a primary disease of the pulmonary vessels.
4. In infancy, a ventricular septal defect may be indistinguishable from a patent ductus arteriosus.
5. The axiom "The louder the murmur, the smaller the defect" does not always apply.
6. The recognition of the diastolic murmur of aortic insufficiency, in the presence of classic findings of ventricular septal defect, should make a supracristal variety very suspect.
7. The supracristal ventricular septal defect occurs more commonly in patients of Asian extraction.
8. The supracristal ventricular septal defect is also known as a "doubly committed ventricular septal defect."

3

Patent Ductus Arteriosus

EMBRYOLOGY

Between the fifth and seventh weeks of gestation, the aortic arch system develops (Fig 3–1). This begins as six paired arches proliferating from the apex of the truncus arteriosus. The sixth, or pulmonary, arch gives off a branch that grows toward the developing lung. On the right side, the proximal portion becomes the proximal portion of the right pulmonary artery and the distal portion disappears. On the left side, the proximal portion becomes the proximal portion of the left pulmonary artery but the distal portion maintains its attachment to the aorta, becoming the ductus arteriosus.

ANATOMY

During fetal life, the ductus arteriosus serves as a functioning connection between the pulmonary artery and the aorta. After birth and with institution of respiration, the partial pressure of oxygen (Po_2) rises and the pulmonary arterioles dilate, each of which influences the ductus arteriosus to close. Ultimately, it will fibrose, becoming the ligamentum arteriosum. Under certain circumstances, however, the ves-

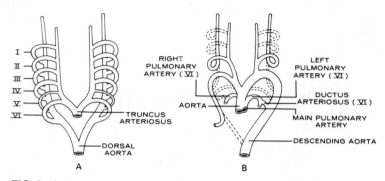

FIG 3-1.

Diagrammatic representation of the development of the aortic arch system as it relates to the ductus arteriosus. Note that the left pulmonary artery and the ductus arteriosus were the embryonic sixth arch.

sel remains open, being called, somewhat redundantly, a patent ductus arteriosus.

HEMODYNAMICS

The patient with a patent ductus arteriosus has an abnormal communication between the aorta with its high pressure and the pulmonary artery with its low pressure, through which a volume of blood flows. This places a volume burden on the lungs and ultimately on the left side of the heart, a situation not dissimilar to the patient with a ventricular septal defect. This is conceptualized in the mnemonic

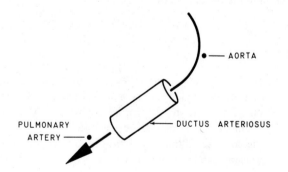

The arrow represents blood flowing from the aorta through the ductus arteriosus into the pulmonary artery. It is also meant to represent the circumstances present in the older infant and young child after the pulmonary vessels have matured and before any supervening secondary pulmonary hypertension has developed. If the flow is followed, its effect on the heart can be demonstrated by the following diagram:

RIGHT ATRIUM →	LEFT ATRIUM → ↑
RIGHT VENTRICLE →	LEFT VENTRICLE → ↑
MAIN PULMONARY ARTERY ↑	AORTA ↑
PULMONARY VESSELS ↑	

The arrows represent alteration in the size of a chamber or a vessel as follows:

→ Unchanged
↑ Increased

Translated to the chest roentgenogram, the pulmonary artery, pulmonary vessels, and the aorta would rather consistently be increased in

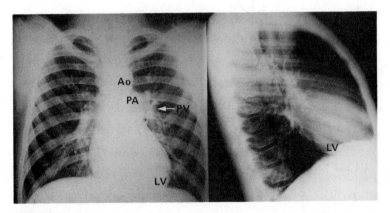

FIG 3–2.
Chest roentgenograms of a 7-year-old patient with patent ductus arteriosus. The salient features are the absence of a significant cardiomegaly, the presence of a full pulmonary artery segment, a prominent aortic knob, and increased pulmonary vessels. Note that on the lateral view the left ventricle is not significantly enlarged. *PA* = pulmonary artery; *Ao* = aorta; *PV* = pulmonary vessels; *LV* = left ventricle.

size. The size of the left atrium and left ventricle would be variable, depending on the magnitude of the shunt (Fig 3–2). If pulmonary hypertension were present, the right ventricle would be enlarged also.

The electrocardiogram (ECG) would be equally variable, ranging from a normal tracing (not shown) to left ventricular hypertrophy (Fig 3–3) or combined ventricular hypertrophy (Fig 3–4). In the face of pulmonary hypertension, right ventricular hypertrophy would be seen (not demonstrated).

Clinical Application

The patient with a patent ductus arteriosus is influenced by changes in the pulmonary vascular bed quite like the patient with a ventricular septal defect. The reader is referred to Chapter 2 for a detailed explanation. It is usual at birth for the resistances in both pulmonary and systemic circuits to be identical. As normal resolution of the pulmonary arterioles takes place, the pulmonary resistance falls, the

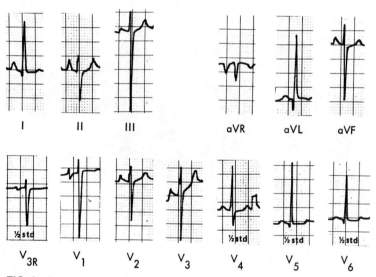

FIG 3–3.
Electrocardiogram of a 7-year-old patient with patent ductus arteriosus showing left ventricular hypertrophy. The salient features are a deep S wave in V_1 and a tall R wave in V_5. In addition, the axis deviation of the bipolar leads is leftward.

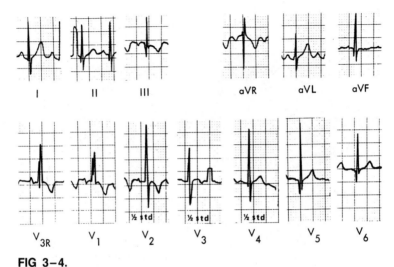

FIG 3–4.

Electrocardiogram of a 6-year-old patient with patent ductus arteriosus showing combined ventricular hypertrophy. The salient features are a dominant R wave in V_1, a dominant R wave in V_5 and V_6, and tall complexes in $V_{2, 3, 4}$.

pulmonary artery pressure drops and a gradient is created between the aorta and the pulmonary artery. Flow then can take place across the ductus. It is common in this age range for there to be a wide pulse pressure in the arterial system, but the diastolic pressure in both the pulmonary artery and the aorta are virtually identical (Fig 3–5). Flow through the ductus then would take place only during systole, and therefore only a systolic murmur would be heard. By the latter half of the first year, with continued maturation in both systemic and pulmonary vessels, a diastolic gradient will also develop, flow will take place in both systole and diastole, and the classic continuous murmur will be heard. The murmurs will occur to the left of the sternum at the second and third interspaces and will transmit not only down the sternum anteriorly but along the course of the pulmonary arteries, being heard quite well in the back. The volume of blood presented to the left side of the heart will cause displacement of the apex laterally and inferiorly. A left ventricular thrust usually will be felt. Increased left ventricular volume may prolong the systolic ejection time, thereby delaying closure of the aortic valve. The right side of the heart will be

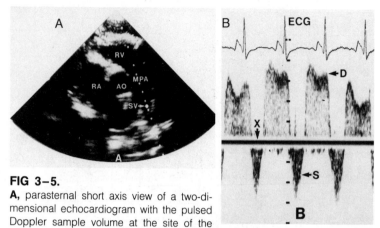

FIG 3-5.
A, parasternal short axis view of a two-dimensional echocardiogram with the pulsed Doppler sample volume at the site of the patent ductus arteriosus. The transducer is at the peak of the triangle. **B,** resulting image of the pulsed Doppler. Note the flow in systole away from the transducer below the baseline and the flow in diastole toward the transducer above the baseline. *RA* = right atrium; *AO* = aorta; *RV* = right ventricle; *MPA* = main pulmonary artery; *SV* = sample volume; *S* = systole; *D* = diastole; *X* = baseline.

affected by variations of venous return, and therefore a normal splitting of the second sound can be anticipated. The intensity of closure of the pulmonary valve will depend on the pulmonary artery pressure and the pulmonary resistances. If the patient is not treated and pulmonary hypertension develops, the pulmonary valve will close with greater intensity and somewhat earlier than normal, creating narrowing of the splitting with an intensification of the pulmonary component.

Extrapolation of this information to the patient now can be attempted. The patient with a patent ductus arteriosus usually will be considered normal at birth. No murmur will be reported. By 2 to 6 weeks of age, flow may begin through the ductus and a systolic murmur will be heard. The left atrium and ventricle will become recipients of a considerable volume overload, leading to two possible courses: First, if the left ventricle cannot accommodate to the load, an increase in diastolic pressure will occur, leading to an increase in left atrial pressure and pulmonary venous engorgement. A cough, dyspnea, tachypnea, and tachycardia may develop, followed by hepatosplenomegaly—the classic symptoms and signs of congestive heart failure.

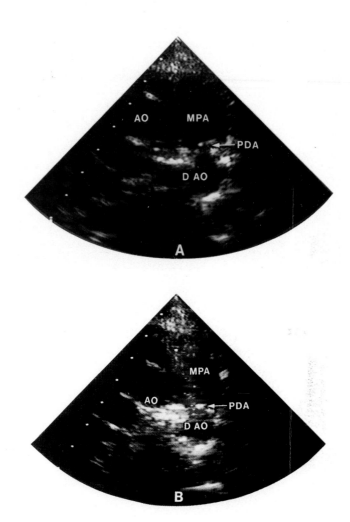

PLATE 3.
A parasternal short-axis view in a patient with a patent ductus arteriosus **(A)** and a similar image with color flow **(B).** The shade of red represents flow through the patent ductus arteriosus into the main pulmonary artery, that flow being toward the transducer at the peak of the triangle. *AO* = aorta at the level of the valves; *MPA* = main pulmonary artery; *D AO* = descending aorta; *PDA* = patent ductus arteriosus.

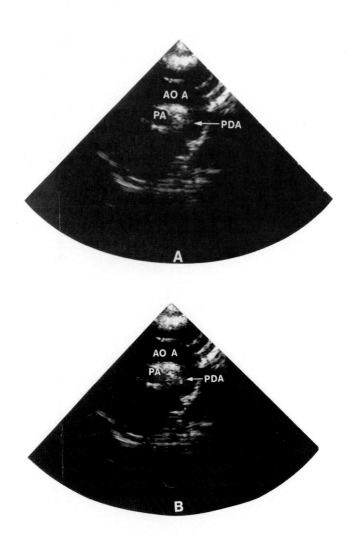

PLATE 4.
A high right sternal border view of an echocardiogram in a patient with a patent ductus arteriosus **(A)** and a similar image with color flow **(B).** The shade of orange represents flow through the ductus itself in **B.** *AO A* = aortic arch; *PA* = pulmonary artery; *PDA* = patent ductus arteriosus.

This infant with a patent ductus arteriosus may be indistinguishable from one with a ventricular septal defect.

Echocardiography can, in most instances, image the ductus itself (Plates 3 and 4). In the parasternal short axis view (see Plate 3) the one most commonly employed, color flow Doppler will show the diastolic flow into the pulmonary artery as a shade of red or orange, which by convention represents flow toward the transducer. Pulsed Doppler can record the normal systolic flow into the pulmonary artery and the abnormal diastolic flow through the ductus into the same pulmonary artery (see Fig 3–5). If needed, and currently rarely so, cardiac catheterization can finally clarify the situation (Table 3–1). It will show an increase in oxygen saturation at the level of the pulmonary artery, thus differentiating it from a ventricular septal defect. In addition, the systolic pressure in the pulmonary artery will be elevated but less than that in the systemic artery, whereas the diastolic pressure in each will be virtually the same (Fig 3–6). Passage of the catheter through the ductus arteriosus into the descending aorta will make the

TABLE 3–1.

Idealized Cardiac Catheterization Data in an Infant Patient With a Patent Ductus Arteriosus*

Site	Pressure (mm Hg)		Oxygen Saturation (%)	
	Normal	Patient	Normal	Patient
Superior vena cava			70	70
Inferior vena cava			74	74
Right atrium	a = 5 v = 4 m = 4	a = 5 v = 4 m = 4	72	72
Right ventricle	25/2	60/5	72	72
Main pulmonary artery	25/12	60/30	72	84
Left atrium	a = 5 v = 7 m = 6	a = 7 v = 9 m = 8	97	97
Left ventricle	90/5	90/5	97	97
Systemic artery	90/50	90/30	97	97

*The salient features are an increase in oxygen saturation in the pulmonary artery, elevation of the systolic pressure in the pulmonary artery, and equal diastolic pressures in the pulmonary artery and the systemic artery. The pressure in the left atrium is slightly elevated also.

Ao 92/32   MPA 64/32   RV 60/4

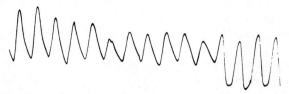

FIG 3–6.
A representative pullback pressure curve in an infant with a patent ductus arteriosus. Note that the diastolic pressure in the aorta and the main pulmonary artery are identical. The systolic pressure in the ventricle is the same as that in the pulmonary artery. *Ao* = aorta; *MPA* = main pulmonary artery; *RV* = right ventricle.

diagnosis absolute (Fig 3–7). Second, if the left ventricle can accommodate to the load, the infant remains asymptomatic and the presence of congenital heart disease is announced merely by the appearance of a systolic murmur. The patient's growth pattern may be reasonable, and ultimately the appearance of a typical continuous murmur permits a clinical diagnosis of a patent ductus arteriosus. Echocardiography can be used, and if it is diagnostic, cardiac catheterization generally can be avoided.

DIFFERENTIAL DIAGNOSIS

The patient with a patent ductus arteriosus must be distinguished from one having a venous hum, a pulmonary arteriovenous fistula, a coronary arteriovenous fistula, a sinus of Valsalva aneurysm, and stenoses of the pulmonary arteries.

Differentiation from the venous hum is most important, because the latter is an innocent phenomenon relating to venous return. It is heard most commonly over the second right interspace but can be present over the second left interspace when a left superior vena cava is present. The murmur tends to disappear with compression of the neck vessels, turning of the head, or assumption of a supine position, each of which alters the quantity and quality of venous return. It is

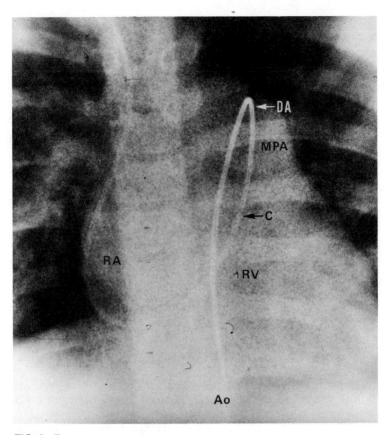

FIG 3-7.
An enlarged photograph of a 35-mm cineangiocardiographic frame showing the classic course of a cardiac catheter in a patient with a patent ductus arteriosus. Note the passage of the catheter from the right side of the heart through the ductus arteriosus into the descending aorta. *RA* = right atrium; *RV* = right ventricle; *MPA* = main pulmonary artery; *DA* = ductus arteriosus; *Ao* = descending aorta; *C* = catheter.

notable that a venous hum virtually always disappears when the patient is lying down, whereas the murmur of a patent ductus arteriosus remains or frequently increases with lying down.

A pulmonary arteriovenous fistula has a comparable continuous murmur but it usually is heard over lung tissue some distance from the heart. If it were present in vessels overlying the heart, further confusion would exist and cardiac catheterization might be needed to effect the diagnosis.

The murmur of a coronary arteriovenous fistula resembles that of the patent ductus but is heard lower on the chest and has a greater diastolic accentuation. Cardiac catheterization, however, almost always will be required to confirm this diagnosis.

The murmur of a sinus of Valsalva aneurysm may be very reminiscent of a patent ductus arteriosus and would require cardiac catheterization for definition.

Stenoses of the pulmonary arteries also may have a continuous murmur, but the diastolic phase frequently is inconsistent. The murmur usually is heard under both clavicles, with transmission through the pulmonary vessels equally to the right and left. Echocardiography can rule out a patent ductus arteriosus, but cardiac catheterization may be necessary to clarify the problem. (This lesion is discussed in greater detail in Chapter 6.)

PEARLS

1. Patent ductus arteriosus occurs more commonly in females than in males.

2. In the infant, bounding posterior tibial and dorsalis pedis pulses help to differentiate a patent ductus arteriosus from a ventricular septal defect.

3. A classic continuous murmur in the first months of life should make one consider other diagnoses before a patent ductus arteriosus.

4. In the premature infant, normal closure of the ductus arteriosus may be delayed beyond the newborn period.

5. The disappearance of the continuous murmur in the supine position supports the diagnosis of a venous hum and is against the diagnosis of a patent ductus arteriosus.

6. Echocardiography with Doppler interrogation has a diagnostic accuracy approaching 100% with this lesion.

4 | Endocardial Cushion Defect

EMBRYOLOGY

Between the fourth and eighth weeks of gestation, the transition from a tubular heart into a four-chambered structure is completed. This is accomplished through four events, namely, septation at the level of the atria (Fig 4–1), septation at the level of the ventricles (see Fig 4–1), proliferation of the endocardial cushions (Fig 4–2), and growth of the bulboconus area (Fig 4–3). The single atrium is divided by growth of a thin wall of tissue—the first septum—that originates in the dorsal wall of the single atrium and proceeds in its growth toward the endocardial cushions. These are concomitantly growing to separate the atria from the ventricles. As the first septum approaches these cushions, the space between the two structures is called the ostium primum, or first hole (see Fig 4–1, A). As it proliferates to seal totally, fenestrations appear in the center of the first septum, leading to a second hole—the ostium secundum. At this time there appears a second thin septum growing to the right of the first—the septum secundum (see Fig 4–1, B). The ultimate balance between proliferation

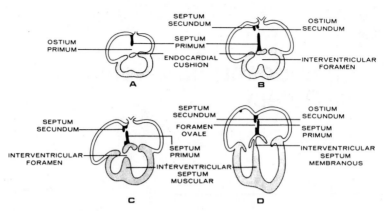

FIG 4–1.
Schematic representation of the formation of the interatrial and interventricular septum. **A,** 30 days; **B,** 33 days; **C,** 37 days; **D,** newborn period. (See text for explanation.) (Modified from Moss AJ, Adams FH [eds]: *Heart Disease in Infants, Children and Adolescents.* Baltimore, Williams & Wilkins Co, 1968, p 16.)

and absorption in these two septa leads to the formation of a hole— the foramen ovale—to be guarded on its left side by a valve (see Fig 4–1, C and D). This arrangement effectively permits blood flow from the right atrium to the left atrium during fetal development. After birth, when left atrial pressure exceeds right atrial pressure, flow in either direction is prevented.

Between the fourth and eighth weeks of gestation, the single ven-

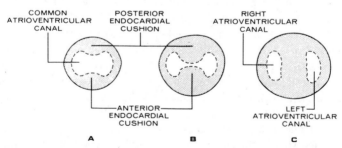

FIG 4–2.
Schematic representation in cross section showing how the endocardial cushions divide the common atrioventricular canal into two. (See text for explanation.)

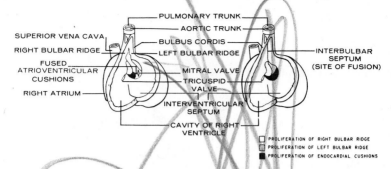

FIG 4-3.
Schematic representation of the role of the bulbus cordis in the formation of the interventricular septum. (See text for explanation.)

tricle is divided by fusion of the membranous portion of the ventricular septum, the endocardial cushions, and the bulbus cordis (the proximal portion of the truncus arteriosus). The muscular portion of the ventricular septum grows cephalad as each ventricular chamber enlarges, eventually meeting with the right and left ridges of the bulbus cordis. The right ridge fuses with the tricuspid valve and the endocardial cushion, thus separating the pulmonary valve from the tricuspid valve. The left ridge fuses with a ridge of the interventricular septum, leaving the aortic ring in continuity with the mitral ring. The endocardial cushions (see Fig 4-2) are concomitantly developing and ultimately fuse with the bulbar ridges (see Fig 4-3) and the muscular portion of the septum. The final closure and separation of the two ventricles are made by the fibrous tissue of the membranous portion of the interventricular septum (see Fig 4-1).

ANATOMY

If the endocardial cushions do not fuse, the atrioventricular valves—tricuspid and mitral—cannot develop properly. In addition, the lower portion of the interatrial septum and the upper portion of the interventricular septum will be deficient and will be unable to meet with the endocardial cushions. This will result in a large central hole

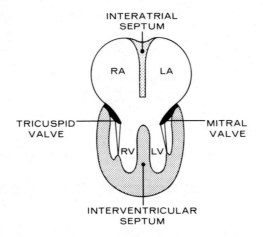

FIG 4–4.
Schematic representation of the anatomy in a complete endocardial cushion defect. The salient feature is a large central hole. (See text for explanation.) *RA* = right atrium; *RV* = right ventricle; *LA* = left atrium; *LV* = left ventricle.

and free communication among all four chambers—the complete form of an endocardial cushion defect (Fig 4–4). Endocardial cushion defects have been classified as partial, intermediate, and complete. The first is an ostium primum defect and is discussed in Chapter 1. The transitional form has partial fusion of the endocardial cushions, resulting in variable abnormalities of the atrioventricular valves, and is not discussed. It is the purpose of this chapter to deal only with the complete form.

HEMODYNAMICS

The patient with an endocardial cushion defect has the potential for blood flow between any of the four chambers of the heart. This flow is dependent on the relative resistances of the pulmonary and systemic circuits, the pressures within the two ventricular chambers, and the relative compliance of all the chambers. This concept is shown in the mnemonic

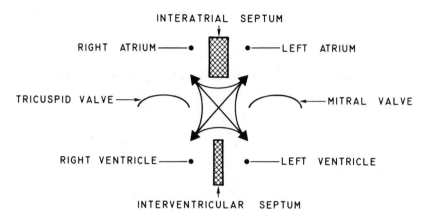

If the blood is followed with the mnemonic in mind, the effect on the various chambers and vessels of the heart can be demonstrated by the following diagram:

RIGHT ATRIUM ↑	LEFT ATRIUM ↑
RIGHT VENTRICLE ↑	LEFT VENTRICLE ↑
MAIN PULMONARY ARTERY ↑	AORTA →
PULMONARY VESSELS ↑	

The arrows represent alteration in the size of a chamber or a vessel as follows:

→ Unchanged
↑ Increased

This information can be translated to the chest roentgenogram, where one would expect to find gross cardiomegaly, enlargement of all four chambers, and increased vascular markings (Fig 4–5). The electrocardiogram (ECG) is generally interpreted as showing right ventricular hypertrophy or combined ventricular hypertrophy. Combined atrial hypertrophy is also frequently seen. The frontal-plane QRS forces would be directed in a counterclockwise fashion, with the initial deflection being rightward and then leftward and superiorly, producing left axis deviation as expressed by the presence of a Q wave in leads I and aVL and a deep S wave in lead aVF (Fig 4–6).

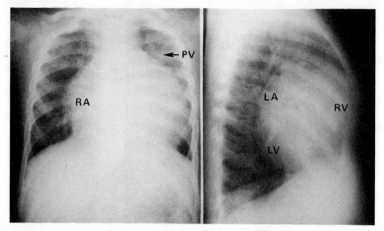

FIG 4–5.
Chest roentgenograms of a patient with an endocardial cushion defect. Note the gross cardiomegaly, with enlargement of all four intercardiac chambers. The pulmonary vessels are increased. RA = right atrium; RV = right ventricle; LA = left atrium; LV = left ventricle; PV = pulmonary vessels.

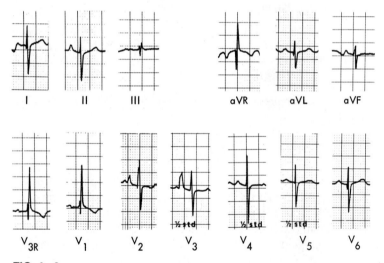

FIG 4–6.
Electrocardiogram of a patient with an endocardial cushion defect. The salient features are a Q wave in leads I and aVL and a deep S wave in lead aVF, which is interpretable as left axis deviation with a counterclockwise inscription of the QRS forces. Note also a tall R' in lead V_1, a deep S in lead V_6, and tall complexes in leads $V_{3, 4, 5}$, which are interpretable as right ventricular hypertrophy with probable coexisting left ventricular hypertrophy.

CLINICAL APPLICATION

It has been suggested that at this point there is potential flow between any of the cardiac chambers at any one time. In addition, pulmonary hypertension of a marked degree is rather consistently present. These two facts influence the clinical picture. Growth is poor, respiratory tract infections are common, and congestive heart failure is frequent. The gross cardiomegaly will cause the left side of the chest to be prominent, and the specific chamber enlargement will be responsible for a right ventricular heave and a left ventricular thrust. In the presence of pulmonary hypertension, intensified closure of the pulmonary valve will be palpable as a tap high on the left side of the chest. All peripheral pulses will be palpable and not unusual. The presence of mitral and tricuspid insufficiency, atrial septal defect, and a ventric-

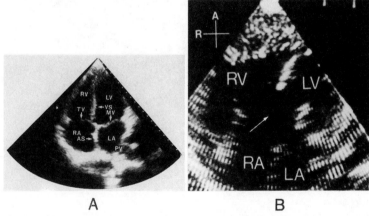

A   B

FIG 4–7.
Apical four-chamber view of an echocardiogram in a normal patient **(A)** and in a patient with a complete endocardial cushion defect **(B).** Image in **B** is taken in diastole. *Arrow* point to echo-free space showing communication between and among all four chambers. *A* = anterior; *R* = right; *RV* = right ventricle; *TV* = tricuspid valve; *RA* = right atrium; *LA* = left atrium; *MV* = mitral valve; *LV* = left ventricle; *RPV* = right pulmonary vein; *LPV* = left pulmonary vein; *MB* = moderator band. (From Silverman NH, Snider AR: *Two-Dimensional Echocardiography in Congenital Heart Disease.* Norwalk, Conn, Appleton-Century-Crofts, 1982, p 87. Used by permission.)

ular septal defect would prompt one to anticipate murmurs representing any or all of these phenomena. This may indeed be the case, but quite often the clinical situation is one of balanced intracardiac dynamics and minimal abnormal shunting, resulting in virtually no murmurs. The presence of pulmonary hypertension is heralded by a single or closely duplicated second sound, with the pulmonary component being significantly increased in intensity. (The latter is the auscultatory equivalent of the pulmonary closure tap.)

The patient may be suspected of having a complete endocardial cushion defect if he or she has poor growth and development, prominence of the left side of the chest, variable murmurs or none at all, an increased pulmonary component of the second sound, gross cardiomegaly on chest roentgenogram with increased vascular markings, and

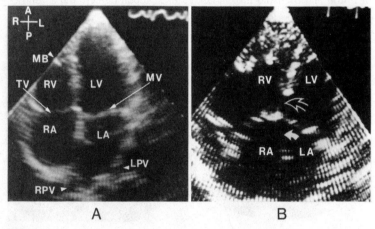

FIG 4–8.
Apical four-chamber view of an echocardiogram in a normal patient **(A)** and in a patient with a complete endocardial cushion defect **(B).** In **B,** the image is in systole with the mitral valve *(MV)* and the tricuspid valve *(TV)* closed. Note *white arrow* pointing to the echo-free space low in the atrial septum and *black arrow* pointing to the echo-free space high in the ventricular septum in **B.** *RV* = right ventricle; *RA* = right atrium; *LA* = left atrium; *LV* = left ventricle; *RPV* = right pulmonary vein; *LPV* = left pulmonary vein; *MB* = moderator band. (From Silverman NH, Snider AR: *Two-Dimensional Echocardiography in Congenital Heart Disease.* Norwalk, Conn, Appleton-Century-Crofts, 1982, p 87. Used by permission.)

an ECG with an abnormal leftward axis and right ventricular or biventricular hypertrophy.

The echocardiogram has evolved as an exquisite tool, permitting noninvasive definition of the various forms of endocardial cushion defects. When it is viewed in real time (actual motion), the insertion of the common or bridging arterioventricular valve at the same level of the crux of the septum can be appreciated. In addition, the insertion of the chordae tendineae of both the right- and left-sided components of the common arterioventricular valve can be accurately identified. In addition, the transitional forms can better be defined by this modality than cardiac catheterization. The illustrations, however, relate only to the complete form (Figs 4–7 and 4–8). The dynamics of the diagnosis can be further elaborated on with cardiac catheterization. This would show that the catheter is able to pass into all four chambers, but in a bizarre manner, such as from the right atrium directly to the left ventricle, with bidirectional intracardiac shunting and systemic pressures in the right ventricle and pulmonary artery (Table 4–1).

TABLE 4–1.

Idealized Cardiac Catheterization Data in an Infant With an Endocardial Cushion Defect*

Site	Pressure (mm Hg) Normal	Pressure (mm Hg) Patient	Oxygen Saturation (%) Normal	Oxygen Saturation (%) Patient
Superior vena cava			70	65
Inferior vena cava			74	70
Right atrium	a = 5 v = 3 m = 4	a = 10 v = 10 m = 9	72	75
Right ventricle	25/2	100/7	72	80
Main pulmonary artery	25/12	100/50	72	80
Pulmonary vein	a = 6 v = 8 m = 7	a = 8 v = 10 m = 9	97	97
Left atrium	a = 5 v = 7 m = 6	a = 8 v = 10 m = 8	97	86
Left ventricle	100/5	100/5	97	82
Systemic artery	100/75	100/75	97	82

*The salient features are an increase in oxygen saturation at the right atrium, a further increase at the right ventricle, a decrease in oxygen saturation at the left atrium, and a further decrease at the level of the left ventricle. The pressures in the right ventricle and the pulmonary artery are systemic in height, whereas those in each atrium are slightly elevated.

DIFFERENTIAL DIAGNOSIS

The patient with a complete endocardial cushion defect must be differentiated from one having pulmonary hypertension with any other lesion. This would include such lesions as a ventricular septal defect with pulmonary hypertension (the Eisenmenger complex), an ostium primum type of an atrial septal defect, a patent ductus arteriosus in an infant, and a type I, II, III truncus arteriosus. The ECG will be of major help in making the correct diagnosis. On occasion a patient with a ventricular septal defect will have an ECG with left axis deviation, which will be confusing; in this circumstance, the combined use of echocardiography and cardiac catheterization will clarify the confusion.

PEARLS

1. The complete form of endocardial cushion defect is the most common cardiac anomaly seen in patients with Down syndrome.

2. Early and unremitting pulmonary hypertension, with the possibility of obstructive pulmonary vascular disease by 1 year of age, is to be expected.

3. There is no sex preference for the lesion.

4. The terms atrioventricular canal and endocardial cushion defect are synonymous and interchangeable.

5. The term canal-type ventricular septal defect refers to a posteriorly placed ventricular septal defect as seen in an atrioventricular canal. It retains the dynamics of a straightforward ventricular septal defect but generally has a leftward axis on the ECG.

6. The term atrioventricular septal defect is being proposed as new nomenclature.

PART II

Obstructive Lesions

5 | Aortic Stenosis and Other Lesions Obstructive to Left Ventricular Outflow

EMBRYOLOGY

Between the sixth and ninth weeks of gestation, the truncus arteriosus is divided into the aorta and the pulmonary artery. At about the same time, the aortic valves develop. These are formed by proliferation of three tubercles within the lumen of the aorta, which grow toward the midline (Fig 5–1). Where the tubercle joins the wall of the aorta, there is resorption of tissue, followed by further hollowing out of tissue, giving rise to the sinuses of the valve (Fig 5–2). During the seventh week of gestation, the coronary arteries develop.

ANATOMY

Obstruction to left ventricular outflow can occur below the valve in either a fixed discrete or variable muscular form, at the valve itself, or above the valve (Fig 5–3). Although similarities exist among the anatomical varieties, the differences are sufficient to warrant a separate discussion of each. The most common variation is discussed first.

VALVULAR AORTIC STENOSIS

Hemodynamics

The patient with valvular aortic stenosis has an obstruction to left ventricular ejection at the level of the valve, which is demonstrated in the mnemonic

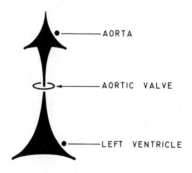

The arrow represents blood flowing from the left ventricle through the obstructed aortic valve into the aorta. The thickened base of the arrow, labeled left ventricle, is meant to represent the increased pressure required to overcome the resistance of the obstructed valve. The head of the arrow represents blood in the ascending aorta. The size of the head is meant to suggest dissipation of energy into the vessel itself. If the blood flow is followed with the mnemonic in mind, the effect on the heart can be demonstrated by the following diagram:

RIGHT ATRIUM →   LEFT ATRIUM →
RIGHT VENTRICLE →   LEFT VENTRICLE ↑
MAIN PULMONARY ARTERY →   ASCENDING AORTA ↑
PULMONARY VESSELS →

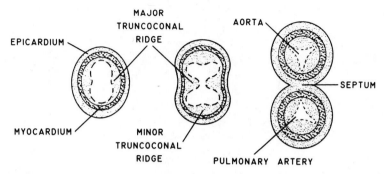

FIG 5–1.
Demonstration of formation of the aortic valves within the aorta. Note the progressive proliferation of the truncoconal ridges. (The pulmonary valves are also demonstrated coincidentally.) (Modified from Moss AJ, Adams FH [eds]: *Heart Disease in Infants, Children and Adolescents.* Baltimore, Williams & Wilkins Co, 1968, p 16.)

The arrows represent alteration in the size of a chamber or a vessel as follows:

$\rightarrow$ Unchanged
↑ Increased

This information can be translated to the chest roentgenogram, where the right side of the heart will be normal, the left ventricle enlarged, and the ascending aorta dilated. Since the effect of the obstruction on the left ventricle is one of muscular hypertrophy rather than

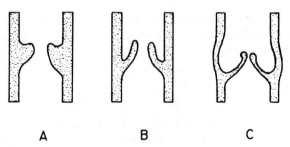

A   B   C

FIG 5–2.
A graphic representation of the proliferation **(A)** and then hollowing out of the tubercles **(B),** giving rise to the completed valve **(C).**

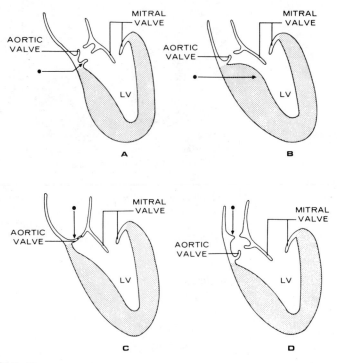

FIG 5–3.
Diagrammatic representation of the various types of obstruction to left ventricular outflow. **A,** discrete subvalvular stenosis; **B,** idiopathic hypertrophic subaortic stenosis; **C,** valvular aortic stenosis; **D,** supravalvular aortic stenosis. *LV* = left ventricle; ●→ = site of obstruction.

dilatation, the overall size of the heart generally is not increased (Fig 5–4). The electrocardiogram (ECG) may show left ventricular hypertrophy but, in fact, may be normal (Fig 5–5).

Clinical Application

The problems presented in this chapter should be collectively considered as "left ventricular outflow tract obstruction." The thinking process from this initial label will require the differentiation of the site of obstruction. Starting with the term "aortic stenosis" almost always

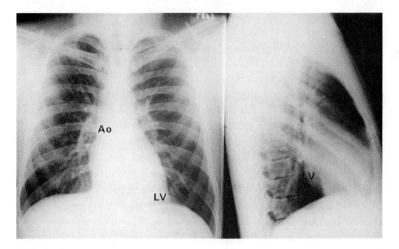

FIG 5–4.
Chest roentgenograms of a child with valvular aortic stenosis. Note the slightly dilated ascending aorta and the left ventricular enlargement. *LV* = left ventricle; *Ao* = aorta.

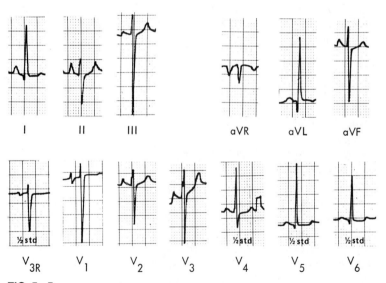

FIG 5–5.
Electrocardiogram of a patient with valvular aortic stenosis. The salient features are the deep S wave in V_1 and tall R waves in $V_{5,6}$, which are interpretable as left ventricular hypertrophy.

directs the individual primarily to the aortic valve and sets the stage for an error in precise diagnosis.

If the patient survives infancy without challenge, he or she generally will grow without difficulty and appear to be normal. The selective hypertrophy of the left ventricle displaces the apex laterally and inferiorly, which can be seen and also felt as a thrust. The first sound will be normal. On opening, the impaired mobility of the aortic valves will cause them to vibrate against the wall of the aorta and will be recognized as an ejection click. Since the aortic valves are located at about the fourth interspace to the left of the sternum, that is where the click will be heard. The murmur follows immediately afterward and is systolic in time, ejection in nature, low-pitched and harsh in quality, and varying in intensity from grade II/VI to grade VI/VI. Even though the murmur is generated as blood passes through the aortic valve, it is heard best at the second interspace to the right of the sternum—the location of maximal intensity of the transmitted sound. Once the intensity reaches or exceeds grade IV/VI, a palpable thrill will accompany the murmur, being present both at the second right interspace and in the suprasternal notch. The thickened nature of the stenotic valve will cause it to close with a less than normal intensity, resulting in a diminished aortic component of the second sound. The more severe the stenosis, the greater the ejection time of the left ventricle and the later the aortic valve close. This will result in a narrowing of the splitting of the second sound. If the stenosis is extraordinarily severe, the aortic valve will, in fact, close after the pulmonary valve and will be recognized as a reversed splitting of the second sound. (This can be identified either clinically or with a phonocardiogram by a narrowing of the splitting with inspiration and a widening of the splitting with expiration.) The intracardiac events will be reflected in the peripheral arterial pulse, which will have a prolonged upstroke with an anacrotic notch, a single sustained peak, and a slow downstroke (Fig 5–6, C). The systemic arterial pressure will have a diminished peak systolic value and a narrow pulse pressure. When the aortic stenosis is caused by abnormalities of a three-leaflet valve, aortic insufficiency is uncommon. When the valve is bicuspid in nature, aortic insufficiency frequently is present and is recognized by the presence of a high-pitched decrescendo diastolic murmur along the left sternal border.

The diagnosis of valvular aortic stenosis can be suspected in a pa-

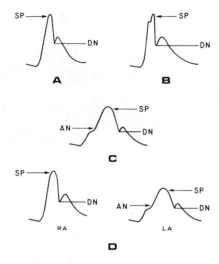

FIG 5–6.
Diagrammatic representation of the various types of peripheral arterial pulse curves in the various forms of obstruction to left ventricular outflow. **A,** normal; **B,** idiopathic hypertrophic subaortic stenosis; **C,** valvular aortic stenosis; **D,** supravalvular aortic stenosis, with *RA* being the right arm and *LA* being the left arm. *AN* = anacrotic notch; *SP* = systolic peak; *DN* = dicrotic notch. (See text for explanation.)

tient, generally a male, who has a small peripheral pulse with a delayed upstroke, a narrow pulse pressure, a left ventricular thrust, a systolic ejection click followed by a systolic ejection murmur, and a palpable thrill at the second right interspace or in the suprasternal notch. The chest roentgenogram would show left ventricular enlargement and a dilated ascending aorta. The ECG might show left ventricular hypertrophy.

If the aortic valve is very severely stenosed, the challenge to the patient is immediate and presents its own unique clinical picture. The infant, usually a male, will be in heart failure with the classic signs of tachypnea, tachycardia, and hepatomegaly. It must be remembered that the anatomical location of the aortic valve is at about the fourth interspace to the left of the sternum. In the infant, the murmur generated by turbulent flow through the stenotic orifice is not only generated at but often is heard best at that location. As such, it may be con-

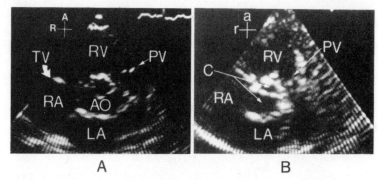

FIG 5–7.
Parasternal short-axis view of an echocardiogram in a normal patient **(A)** and in a patient with a bicuspid aortic valve **(B).** Note the *(arrows)* in **B** pointing to the asymmetric size of the two aortic cusps. *A* = anterior; *R* = right; *RV* = right ventricle; *TV* = tricuspid valve; *RA* = right atrium; *LA* = left atrium; *AO* = aorta; *PV* = pulmonary valve; *c* = cusps. (From Silverman NH, Snider AR: *Two-Dimensional Echocardiography in Congenital Heart Disease.* Norwalk, Conn, Appleton-Century-Crofts, 1982, p 104. Used by permission.)

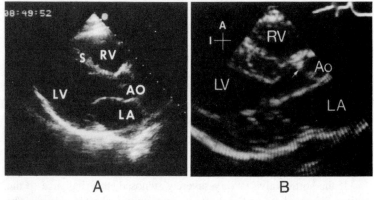

FIG 5–8.
Long-axis view of an echocardiogram in a normal patient **(A)** and in a patient with valvular aortic stenosis **(B).** Note *arrow* in **B** pointing to the thickened aortic valve. *A* = anterior; *I* = inferior; *RV* = right ventricle; *S* = septum; *LV* = left ventricle; *LA* = left atrium; *Ao* = aorta. (From Silverman NH, Snider AR: *Two-Dimensional Echocardiography in Congenital Heart Disease.* Norwalk, Conn, Appleton-Century-Crofts, 1982, p 101. Used by permission.)

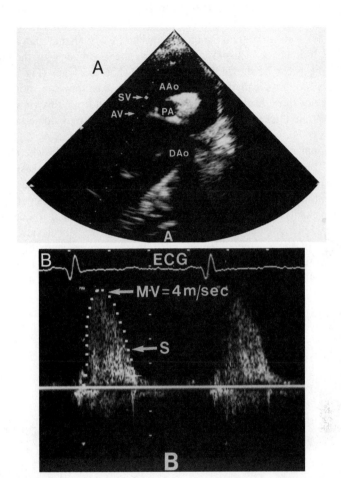

FIG 5–9.
A, a high right parasternal view of a two-dimensional echocardiogram with the sample volume in the ascending aorta above the aortic valve. The transducer is at the peak of the triangle. **B,** the resulting continuous wave image. The maximum velocity of 4 m/sec is toward the transducer and therefore is above the baseline (see text). *AV* = aortic valve; *AAo* = ascending aorta; *DAo* = descending aorta; *PA* = pulmonary artery; *SV* = sample volume; *MV* = maximum velocity; S = systole.

fused with the murmur caused by flow through a ventricular septal defect.

The echocardiogram is quite capable of visualizing the aortic valve. If it has a bicuspid configuration, the asymmetry of the two valve cusps can be shown in the parasternal short-axis view (Fig 5–7). If there are three leaflets, the parasternal long-axis view can show the opening of those leaflets (Fig 5–8). If seen in real time, this view will demonstrate thickened leaflets that move poorly and may dome in systole.

Doppler interrogation has now surfaced as a modality whereby a gradient across a stenotic aortic valve can be estimated noninvasively. If the modified Bernoulli formula (4 × maximum velocity^2) is used, a gradient can be mathematically determined from a recorded maximum velocity. These observations can be made from either imaging in the high right parasternal view (Fig 5–9) or the apical view (Fig 5–10). In the example demonstrated in the figures, regardless of the imaging location, the maximum velocity registered is approximately 4.0 cm/sec. Therefore, applying the formula 4 × 4.0 cm/

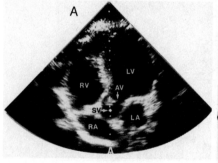

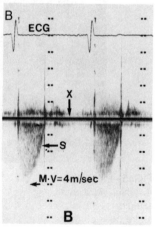

FIG 5–10.
A, an apical four-chamber view of a two-dimensional echocardiogram with the sample volume in the ascending aorta above the aortic valve. The transducer is at the peak of the triangle. **B,** the resultant continuous wave Doppler image. Note the maximum velocity of 4 m/sec below the baseline, which is away from the transducer (see text). *RA* = right atrium; *RV* = right ventricle; *LA* = left atrium; *LV* = left ventricle; *AV* = aortic valve; *SV* = sample volume; *X* = baseline; *S* = systole; *MV* = maximum velocity.

TABLE 5–1.

Idealized Cardiac Catheterization Data in a Child With Valvular Aortic Stenosis*

Site	Pressure (mm Hg)		Oxygen Saturation (%)	
	Normal	Patient	Normal	Patient
Superior vena cava			70	70
Inferior vena cava			74	74
Right atrium	a = 5 v = 4 m = 4	a = 5 v = 4 m = 4	72	72
Right ventricle	25/2	25/2	72	72
Main pulmonary artery	25/12	25/12	72	72
Left ventricle	110/5	160/10	97	97
Aorta	110/80	90/70	97	97

*The salient features are elevated pressures in the left ventricle and diminished pressures with a narrow pulse pressure in the aorta. The oxygen saturations are normal.

sec^2 would calculate to an estimated gradient of approximately 64 mm Hg.

The diagnosis can be confirmed with cardiac catheterization, during which one would find an elevated left ventricular systolic pressure with a diminished aortic systolic pressure, the gradient occurring at the valve. Oxygen saturations will be normal (Table 5–1). Cineangiocardiography will demonstrate the nature of the obstructed valve.

IDIOPATHIC HYPERTROPHIC SUBAORTIC STENOSIS

Hemodynamics

The obstruction to left ventricular outflow is related to the asymmetric enlargement of the left side of the ventricular septum and the proximity of the anterior leaflet of the mitral valve to that septal hypertrophy. It must be clearly understood that this lesion is a dynamic one and that the obstruction is variable, which results in physical findings that are equally variable. The concept of the obstruction is demonstrated in the mnemonic

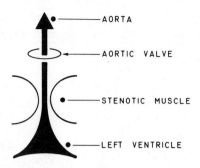

The arrow represents blood flowing from the left ventricle past the obstructive muscle through a normal aortic valve into the aorta. The thickened base of the arrow represents the increased pressure required to overcome the resistance offered by the stenotic muscle. The head of the arrow represents the blood in the aorta and is not enlarged, suggesting the absence of extraordinary pressure in that vessel. If the blood flow is followed with the mnemonic in mind, the effect on the heart can be shown in the following diagram:

RIGHT ATRIUM →   LEFT ATRIUM →
RIGHT VENTRICLE →   LEFT VENTRICLE ↑
MAIN PULMONARY ARTERY →   ASCENDING AORTA →
PULMONARY VESSELS →

The arrows are meant to represent alteration in a chamber or vessel as follows:

→ Unchanged
↑ Increased

This information can be translated to the chest roentgenogram, where the right side of the heart will be normal, the left ventricle will be enlarged, but the ascending aorta will not be dilated. There generally is cardiomegaly (Fig 5–11). If the ECG shows left ventricular hypertrophy (and it may not), Figure 5–5 would be representative.

Clinical Application

It must be emphasized that the area of obstruction is subvalvular and that the valves themselves are normal. As the left ventricle en-

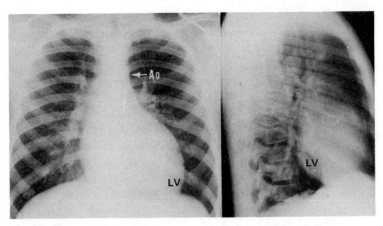

FIG 5-11.
Chest roentgenograms of a child with idiopathic hypertrophic subaortic stenosis. Note the cardiac enlargement with specific left ventricular enlargement and the absence of dilatation of the ascending aorta. *LV* = left ventricle; *Ao* = aorta.

larges, the apex will be displaced laterally and inferiorly and will be visible and also felt as a thrust. With systolic contraction, the obstruction is met and a midsystolic ejection murmur results. Because the obstruction is below the valve, this murmur generally is heard near the apex. Occasionally transmission of the murmur into the ascending aorta may take place and be heard at the second interspace to the right of the sternum, but it rarely transmits into the neck vessels. If the murmur is of sufficient intensity, a thrill will accompany it and be felt near the apex. The aortic valves being normal, an ejection click generally is not heard, the second sound is normal, and aortic insufficiency is not present.

The dynamic nature of this entity is further demonstrated by the variability of the findings when the patient is challenged with certain physiologic modalities. Amyl nitrite, which decreases systemic blood pressure, and the Valsalva maneuver, which decreases venous return, each increases the gradient and thereby increases the intensity of the murmur. Contrariwise, a nonpharmacologic event, such as clenching of the fists or squatting, elevates systemic blood pressure, decreases the gradient and causes a diminution of the murmur.

The systolic events are translated into an unusual peripheral pulse curve in which there is an immediate initial rapid upstroke, followed by a second upstroke shortly thereafter. The pulse pressure tends to be normal (see Fig 5–6, B).

The diagnosis of idiopathic hypertrophic subaortic stenosis can be suspected in a patient, generally an adolescent male, who has a rapid upstroke of his arterial pulse, a left ventricular thrust, the absence of a systolic ejection click, but the presence of a systolic ejection murmur, loudest near the apex with virtually no transmission into the neck, and which increases in intensity with the Valsalva maneuver and decreases in intensity with clenching of the fists or squatting. The chest roentgenogram would show cardiomegaly with left ventricular enlargement, and the ECG might show left ventricular hypertrophy. Echocardiography may demonstrate the apposition of the anterior leaflet of the mitral valve to the left side of the ventricular septum. Confirmation can be obtained with cardiac catheterization, during which one finds elevated left ventricular pressure near the apex but diminished left ventricular pressure in the subvalvular area and in the ascending aorta (Table

TABLE 5–2.

Idealized Cardiac Catheterization Data in a Child With Idiopathic Hypertrophic Subaortic Stenosis*

Site	Pressure (mm Hg) Normal	Pressure (mm Hg) Patient	Oxygen Saturation (%) Normal	Oxygen Saturation (%) Patient
Superior vena cava			70	70
Inferior vena cava			74	74
Right atrium	a = 5 v = 4 m = 5	a = 5 v = 4 m = 5	72	72
Right ventricle	25/2	25/2	72	72
Main pulmonary artery	25/12	25/12	72	72
Left ventricle	110/5	170/7	97	97
Left ventricle, subvalvular	110/5	110/5	97	97
Aorta	110/80	110/75	97	97

*The salient features are an increase in pressure in the left ventricle and a decrease in pressure in the subvalvular area of the left ventricle and the aorta. The oxygen saturations are normal.

5–2). Cineangiocardiography will demonstrate the abnormality of the left ventricular outflow tract.

DISCRETE SUBVALVULAR STENOSIS

The fibrous ring with the narrowed central orifice that sits just below the normal aortic valves results in physical findings that are quite similar to those seen in valvular aortic stenosis. The chest is symmetric. With enlargement of the left ventricle, there is displacement of the apex laterally and inferiorly, which can be seen and also felt as a thrust. A systolic ejection murmur generally will be heard at the second interspace to the right of the sternum, with transmission out the great vessels; if loud enough, it will be accompanied by a thrill. Should the fibrous ring be some distance below the valve, the murmur may be heard best along the middle to lower left sternal border. The aortic valves remain normal, and, therefore, an ejection click generally is not present. The ascending aorta is protected somewhat from the force of ejection through the ring by the normal aortic valves, and secondary dilatation generally does not occur.

Aortic insufficiency, as recognized by a decrescendo diastolic murmur at the third and fourth interspaces to the left of the sternum, is a very common finding. Reasons for this are not abundantly clear. However, it has been suggested that the fibrous ring may interfere with the support structure of the annulus. In addition, the jet created by the ring may cause deterioration of the valve apparatus or the leaflets themselves. Regardless of the etiology, however, progressive aortic insufficiency, with time, is to be expected in a great majority of patients.

The diagnosis of discrete subvalvular stenosis can be suspected in a patient who has physical findings rather consistent with valvular aortic stenosis but who is missing an ejection click and has aortic insufficiency.

The echocardiogram can nicely visualize a density below normal aortic valves, identifying it as a subvalvular membrane (Fig 5–12). Doppler interrogation using the same principles as discussed on page 62 can be used to estimate the gradient across the obstructing membrane. In the presence of aortic insufficiency, the increased volume

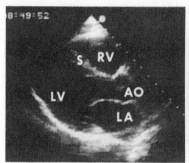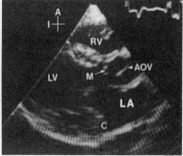

FIG 5-12.
Parasternal long-axis view of an echocardiogram in a normal patient **(A)** and in a patient with a membranous-type subaortic stenosis **(B)**. Note in **B** the *white arrow* pointing to membrane *(M)* in the area below the aortic valve *(AOV)*. *A* = anterior; *I* = inferior; *RV* = right ventricle; *S* = septum; *LV* = left ventricle; *LA* = left atrium; *C* = coronary sinus; *AO* = aorta. (From Silverman NH, Snider AR: *Two-Dimensional Echocardiography in Congenital Heart Disease.* Norwalk, Conn, Appleton-Century-Crofts, 1982, p 106. Used by permission.)

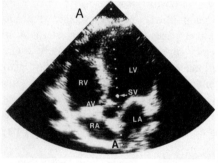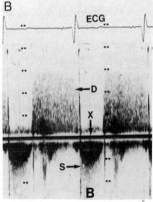

FIG 5-13.
A, an apical four-chamber view of a two-dimensional echocardiogram in a patient with aortic insufficiency. The pulsed Doppler sample volume is in the outflow tract of the left ventricle below the aortic valve. The transducer is at the peak of the triangle. **B,** the resulting image of the pulsed Doppler. Note the dominant flow above the baseline in diastole, which is toward the transducer, and the flow below the baseline in systole, which is away from the transducer. *RA* = right atrium; *RV* = right ventricle; *LA* = left atrium; *LV* = left ventricle; *AV* = aortic valve; *SV* = sample volume; *D* = diastole; *X* = baseline; *S* = systole.

presented to the left ventricle, which it then must eject in systole, will cause the Doppler interrogation to overestimate the gradient.

If aortic insufficiency is present, an apical four-chamber view with the sample volume placed in the outflow tract of the left ventricle can confirm it by recording turbulence in diastole (Fig 5–13). If indicated, cardiac catheterization can then confirm this finding and demonstrate the gradient resulting from the subvalvular stenosis. Cineangiocardiography will further delineate the fixed subvalvular ring. This is not demonstrated.

SUPRAVALVULAR STENOSIS

Supravalvular stenosis is an uncommon form of left ventricular outflow obstruction and is presented for completeness. When present, it is commonly seen as part of a syndrome that includes mental retardation and elfin facies. Hypercalcemia and peripheral pulmonary artery stenoses frequently are also present.

The peripheral pulses are of particular interest in that the right radial pulse may be virtually normal, whereas the left radial pulse will show a delayed upstroke, a prolonged peaking, and a somewhat delayed downstroke. Reasons for this difference are not clear but may relate to the preferential flow of blood through the obstruction into the right-sided vessels, with subsequent dissipation of forces by the time the left brachial artery is reached. The first sound remains normal. An ejection click is not heard. Shortly after the opening of the normal aortic valves, the area of obstruction is encountered and an ejection systolic murmur, grade II/VI or louder, harsh in quality and low in pitch, will be generated. This murmur will be transmitted along the arterial vessels but preferentially into the right-sided rather than the left-sided arteries. If the murmur is of sufficient intensity, a thrill will be palpable and may be higher in the chest than that seen in valvular stenosis. The valves being normal, closure will be secure, and the diastolic murmur of aortic insufficiency will not be heard.

The diagnosis can be suspected in a patient who has physical findings reminiscent of aortic stenosis but who also has mental retardation and elfin facies. Two-dimensional echocardiography can generally image the area of stenosis above the valve, and as in other forms of left

ventricular outflow tract obstruction, Doppler interrogation can estimate the gradient. If indicated, further data can be obtained with cardiac catheterization, during which the pressures in the left ventricle
and those just distal to the aortic valve would be normal and the pressure in the arch of the aorta would be diminished. Cineangiocardiography will visually demonstrate the narrowing within the aorta itself.
These events are not demonstrated.

DIFFERENTIAL DIAGNOSIS

The location of the murmur in the newborn would immediately
raise the question of a ventricular septal defect, but it is unusual for
the murmur of a ventricular septal defect to be present in the newborn
nursery. If so, it generally is caused by a small, muscular defect with
little physiologic challenges. Pulse rates would be normal, and the infant would not be in distress. Echocardiography with Doppler interrogation, including color flow, will be useful in effecting the differential
diagnosis.

PEARLS

1. Aortic stenosis is more common in males than in females.
2. Although reverse splitting of the second sound can be expected in
very severe aortic stenosis, it also can be seen with a left bundle-branch
block.
3. The physical findings in the infant may be different from those in
the child.
4. The degree of gradient across the aortic valve cannot always be
suspected on the basis of the amount of left ventricular hypertrophy on
the ECG.
5. The presence of a systolic ejection click strongly suggests that
the obstruction is at the valve.
6. A bicuspid aortic valve is seen quite commonly in patients with
coarctation of the aorta.
7. Think "left ventricular outflow tract obstruction" when considering
aortic stenosis, because it will instinctively urge you to consider all of
the sites of potential obstruction.

6 | Pulmonary Stenosis and Other Lesions Obstructive to Right Ventricular Outflow

EMBRYOLOGY

Between the sixth and ninth weeks of gestation, concomitant with the development of the truncus arteriosus, the pulmonary valve develops. It is formed by enlargement of three tubercles within the lumen of the pulmonary artery (Fig 6–1). The tubercles grow toward the midline and are thinned by resorption of tissue. There is additional hollowing out of tissue at the superior portion of the tubercle at its junction with the wall of the pulmonary artery, giving rise to the sinuses of the valve (Fig 6–2).

Slightly before the development of the pulmonary valves, the infundibulum of the right ventricle is being formed from the proximal portion of the bulbus cordis.

At about the same time—the fifth to the seventh week of gestation—the aortic arch system is differentiating. The sixth arch becomes the distal portion of the pulmonary artery. Distally, it connects to the smaller pulmonary arteries, which develop from the pulmonary vascular plexus, and proximally it connects to the main pulmonary artery.

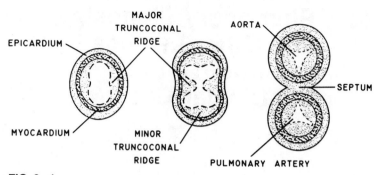

EPICARDIUM

MAJOR
TRUNCOCONAL
RIDGE

AORTA

MYOCARDIUM

MINOR
TRUNCOCONAL
RIDGE

SEPTUM

PULMONARY ARTERY

FIG 6–1.
Demonstration of formation of the pulmonary valves within the pulmonary artery. Note the progressive proliferation of the truncoconal ridges. (The aortic valves are also demonstrated coincidentally.) (Modified from Moss AJ, Adams FH [eds]: *Heart Disease in Infants, Children and Adolescents.* Baltimore, Williams & Wilkins Co, 1968, p 16.)

ANATOMY

Failure of normal development of the tissue-thin three leaflets of the pulmonary valve will result in an abnormality of that valve. The valve may have only two leaflets that may be fused at their common commissures. Three leaflets may develop but may be thickened and partially fused at their commissures or totally fused, with no semblance of commissures, giving a conelike, tunnel-shaped valve resem-

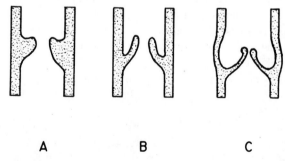

A   B   C

FIG 6–2.
A graphic representation of the proliferation **(A)** and then hollowing out of the tubercles **(B),** giving rise to the completed valve **(C).**

bling, somewhat, the mouth of a fish. Being able to picture the narrow orifice of either two or three leaflets, which grossly restricts valve motion, will aid in the understanding of the dynamics of the lesion.

If there is insufficient resorption of tissue in the bulbus cordis, an area of infundibular hypertrophy will result. In addition, abnormal bands of muscle may be laid down within the body of the right ventricle.

Last, in the development of the peripheral pulmonary arteries, the hollowing out of those vessels may be interfered with, giving rise to multiple areas of stenosis.

HEMODYNAMICS

A common denominator in each of these lesions, regardless of its specific location, is an obstruction to right ventricular systolic ejection. This effectively presents a pressure burden—enormous at times—on the right ventricle. This is conceptualized in the following mnemonic, which demonstrates an obstruction at the pulmonary valve but is applicable in principle, regardless of the location of the obstruction.

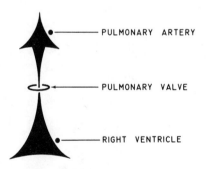

The arrow represents blood flowing from the right ventricle through the narrowed valve into the pulmonary artery. The tip of the arrow has passed the obstructed valve, dissipating its energy into the pulmonary artery. The base of the arrow represents the force required to overcome the area of obstruction.

If the blood flow is followed with the mnemonic in mind, the effect on the size of chambers and vessels of the heart can be demonstrated by the following diagram:

RIGHT ATRIUM → ↑	LEFT ATRIUM →
RIGHT VENTRICLE ↑	LEFT VENTRICLE →
MAIN PULMONARY ARTERY ↑	AORTA →
LEFT PULMONARY ARTERY ↑	
PULMONARY VESSELS →	

The arrows represent alteration in the size of a chamber or a vessel as follows:

→ Unchanged
↑ Increased

In valvular pulmonary stenosis, this effect is directly transferable to the chest roentgenogram. One would expect right ventricular enlargement, main pulmonary artery enlargement, normal pulmonary vascularity, and a normal left side (Fig 6–3). The electrocardiogram (ECG) also would be expected to show right ventricular hypertrophy (Fig 6–4). When severe stenosis is present, right atrial hypertrophy will be seen also.

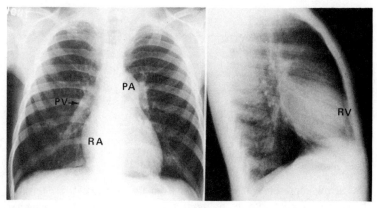

FIG 6–3.
Chest roentgenograms of a patient with valvular pulmonary stenosis. Note the normal right atrium, the enlarged right ventricle impinging on the retrosternal space, and the dilated pulmonary artery. The pulmonary vessels are normal. *RA* = right atrium; *RV* = right ventricle; *PA* = pulmonary artery; *PV* = pulmonary vessels.

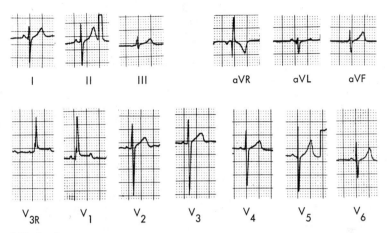

FIG 6–4.
Electrocardiogram of a 4-year-old patient with valvular pulmonary stenosis. The salient features are the dominant S_1 and R/S_{aVF}—right axis deviation. Also present are a dominant R wave in V_1 and S wave in $V_{5,6}$, interpretable as right ventricular hypertrophy. The T wave in V_1 is also upright.

If the obstruction is in the infundibulum, the right ventricular force will be dissipated through the elongated area of obstruction in such a way as to eliminate the abnormal dilatation of the pulmonary artery distal to the valve. On roentgenogram, the pulmonary artery would not be dilated. The ECG would continue to show the abnormal right-sided work load. This is not demonstrated.

Obstruction within the ventricular chamber itself would reflect in the ECG and chest roentgenogram in a fashion similar to obstruction at the infundibulum.

Stenosis of the peripheral pulmonary arteries will have variable radiographic and ECG findings, depending on the severity and location of the lesions.

CLINICAL APPLICATION

Although the site of obstruction is not critical in understanding certain principles, it does affect the details of clinical interpretation and the precise diagnosis. Therefore, each variety of right ventricular obstruction will be discussed individually.

Valvular Stenosis

Valvular stenosis may be mild to very severe. An estimate as to the severity can be made on the basis of the physical examination. In severe stenosis, the excursion of the valve is most limited and the murmur will begin with the first heart sound, ascending in crescendo throughout most of systole, becoming decrescendo, ending at and obscuring the pulmonary component of the second sound. The murmur will be grade IV/VI or greater, generating a palpable thrill at the second left interspace. It will be transmitted along the pulmonary vessels, so it can be expected to be heard in the back. Ejection time will be delayed, resulting in a delayed closure of the pulmonary valve. The significantly restricted excursion capability of the stenosed valve will diminish the intensity of its closure. This will result in a very widely split second sound with a diminished pulmonary component. The splitting may be recognized only on a pnonocardiogram. A right ventricular lift usually would be felt.

If the stenosis is moderate, the first sound will occur and the valves will open, giving rise to an ejection click, which will be followed promptly by the systolic ejection murmur. This will tend to peak somewhat earlier in systole becoming decrescendo, ending after the aortic component of the second sound but before the pulmonary component. The splitting of the second sound may not be as wide and the intensity of the closure of the pulmonary valve not as diminished.

The relationship between the severity of stenosis, the ejection click, and the ejection murmur now can be applied to mild pulmonary stenosis. The milder the stenosis, the wider will be the interval between the first sound and the ejection click, and the peak of the ejection murmur will be reached earlier, with a decrescendo phase ending either with the aortic closure or before the aortic closure. This concept is described beautifully by Perloff and is shown in Figure 6-5.

The parasternal short-axis view of the two-dimensional echocardiogram can demonstrate the outflow tract of the right ventricle and the pulmonary valve. If pulmonary stenosis is present, the valve will

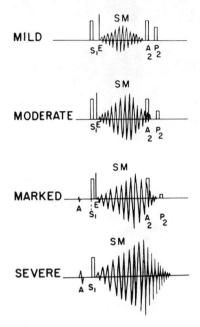

FIG 6–5.
A graphic representation of the relationship between the first sound, the ejection click, the systolic, the aortic, and pulmonic components of the second sound and the appearance of an atrial sound in pulmonary stenosis. (See text for explanation.) S_1 = first sound; E = ejection click; SM = systolic murmur; A_2 = aortic component; P_2 = pulmonic component; A = atrial sound. (Modified from Perloff JK: *The Clinical Recognition of Congenital Heart Disease*. Philadelphia, WB Saunders Co, 1973, p 145.)

be thickened, perhaps domed and the main pulmonary artery dilated (Fig 6–6). If the same parasternal short-axis view is used, an estimate of the gradient across the stenotic valve can be made. With continuous wave Doppler, a maximum velocity can be registered, as in Figure 6–7. The maximum velocity is 4.0 m/sec. If the modified Bernoulli formula ($4 \times$ maximum velocity^2) is used, the gradient can be estimated to be 64 mm Hg. Cardiac catheterization can then be used to delineate the pathology and confirm the estimated gradient and, therefore, degree of severity (Table 6–1). Angiocardiography will show the nature of the stenotic valve and its annulus.

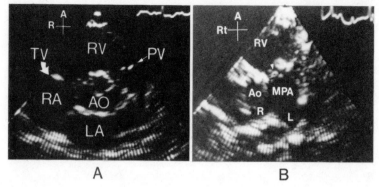

FIG 6–6.
Parasternal short-axis view in a normal patient **(A)** and in a patient with valvular pulmonary stenosis **(B)**. Note *white arrow* in **B** pointing to thickened pulmonary valve and the large main pulmonary artery *(MPA)*. A = anterior; R = right; RV = right ventricle; TV = tricuspid valve; RA = right atrium; LA = left atrium; AO = aorta; PV = pulmonary vein; R = right pulmonary artery; L = left pulmonary artery. (From Silverman NH, Snider AR: *Two-Dimensional Echocardiography in Congenital Heart Disease*. Norwalk, Conn, Appleton-Century-Crofts, 1982, p 113. Used by permission.)

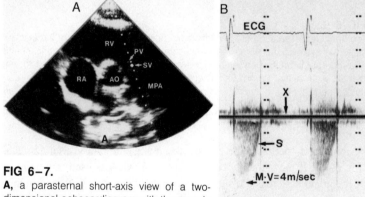

FIG 6–7.
A, a parasternal short-axis view of a two-dimensional echocardiogram with the sample volume in the main pulmonary artery distal to the pulmonary valve. The transducer is at the peak of the triangle. **B,** the resultant continuous wave Doppler image. Note the maximum velocity of 4 m/sec below the baseline, which is away from the transducer (see text). RA = right atrium; RV = right ventricle; PV = pulmonary valve; MPA = main pulmonary artery; AO = aorta, SV = sample volume; X = baseline; S = systole; MV = maximum velocity.

TABLE 6–1.

Idealized Cardiac Catheterization Data in a Child With Valvular
Pulmonary Stenosis*

Site	Pressure (mm Hg)		Oxygen Saturation (%)	
	Normal	Patient	Normal	Patient
Superior vena cava			70	70
Inferior vena cava			74	74
Right atrium	a = 5 v = 3 m = 4	a = 9 v = 6 m = 6	72	72
Right ventricle	25/2	80/4	72	72
Main pulmonary artery	25/12	15/9	72	72
Left pulmonary artery	25/12	15/9	72	72
Systemic artery	120/80	120/80	97	97

*The salient features are an increase in pressure in the right ventricle and a slight decrease in pressure in the pulmonary arteries. There is no change in oxygen saturations.

Malignant Pulmonary Stenosis

An unusual and particularly devastating form of severe valvular pulmonary stenosis occurs in the infant. It is a unique expression of valvular stenosis and is best described as it appears clinically.

At about 6 months of age, the severe stenosis so greatly restricts right ventricular output that acute and sudden right ventricular failure ensues. The resulting increase in end-diastolic pressure causes tricuspid insufficiency and a concomitant increase in right atrial pressure. Dilatation of the right atrium follows, with the foramen ovale becoming incompetent. A right-to-left shunt follows. The previously established systolic ejection murmur diminishes acutely and cyanosis occurs, along with the expected clinical signs of congestive heart failure.

Usually, the diagnosis of pulmonary stenosis has been considered before the acute episode. If not, echocardiography should be able to establish whether a ventricular septal defect and overriding of the aorta are present, which would point to a diagnosis of tetralogy of Fallot. If these findings were absent, and if the pulmonary valve were demonstrated to be thickened and domed, the diagnosis of malignant pulmonary stenosis would be the first choice. Cardiac catheterization and angiocardiography, if indicated, would further confirm the diagnosis. Although this is about the same time that patients with tetralogy of Fallot also become cyanotic, the presence of congestive heart failure strongly supports a diagnosis of pulmonary stenosis with intact septum, in contradistinction to tetralogy of Fallot.

Anomalous Muscle Bundles

These muscle bundles effectively divide the right ventricle into two chambers. The inflow portion near the tricuspid valve would be the high-pressure area, whereas the outflow portion below the pulmonary valve would be the low-pressure area. The valves themselves and the pulmonary artery will be normal. As the ventricle begins systole, the obstruction is encountered immediately; no ejection click is heard, and the murmur will begin with the first sound and end before the second sound. Its location will be lower on the chest, in the vicinity of the third or fourth interspace. The intensity of the murmur will vary with the degree of stenosis, being as small as grade II/VI or as great as grade IV/VI. A thrill will be palpable with the latter. If the obstruction is severe, the proximal portion of the right ventricle will be greatly hypertrophied and will impinge on the retrosternal space. This would cause a bulging of the lower portion of the left precordium. Its contractions would be felt as a right ventricular lift or heave.

The closure of the pulmonary valve may be delayed because of prolongation of right ventricular ejection time. The poststenotic force of blood flow is dissipated in the infundibular area of the right ventricle, which, when combined with normal valve tissue, would give rise to a normal intensity of valvular closure. One then would expect a wide splitting of the second sound, with a normal pulmonary component.

This lesion is not easily differentiated from other forms of right ventricular obstruction, and cardiac catheterization with angiocardiography is necessary to make the differentiation. Pressure tracings will show the differences within the right ventricle, and an angiogram from the right atrium will visually demonstrate the area of obstruction.

Peripheral Pulmonary Artery Stenosis

As implied in this heading, the pulmonary arteries themselves can be stenosed. As demonstrated in Figure 6–8, these areas of stenoses may be single or multiple, localized or diffuse. In all instances, the murmur is a result of turbulence through the obstruction. The point of maximal intensity of the murmur will depend on the location of the obstruction, and the transmission of the murmur will be distal to the obstruction throughout the pulmonary arterial tree. The murmur of the usual multiple peripheral pulmonary artery stenosis is heard at the second interspace, to the left and right of the sternum, and is transmitted well beneath each clavicle, into each axilla and throughout the back. The murmur generally is systolic in time and ejection in character. It is possible, however, for turbulence to occur in both systole and diastole, and a murmur reminiscent of a ductus arteriosus can be heard.

Because the pulmonary valves are normal and the obstruction is distal to them, no ejection click is heard. Since the obstruction will result in a high-pressure area proximal to it but distal to the pulmonary valves, it can be anticipated that normal closure of the valves will occur, but the intensity of the pulmonary component may be increased, depending on the severity of the stenosis.

Although the ECG may show right ventricular hypertrophy, its relationship to the degree of severity is not clearly as accurate as with valvular stenosis. A chest roentgenogram will not be particularly useful in identifying this entity. Cardiac catheterization and angiocardiography, however, will be useful in defining the specific location and nature of the lesions.

Echocardiography has limited use in this lesion. It can image the main and proximal right and left pulmonary arteries effectively. If, however, the stenosis is multiple and beyond the bifurcation, its use is significantly limited.

A patient can be suspected of having an obstruction to right ventricular outflow if he or she is asymptomatic and has prominence of the left side of the chest with a palpable heave, a systolic ejection click at the second interspace to the left of the sternum, a widely duplicated second sound with a diminished pulmonary component, a systolic ejection murmur loudest at the second and third interspaces to the left of the sternum that transmits to the back, and a thrill at the site of the

TYPE I
SINGLE, CENTRAL STENOSIS

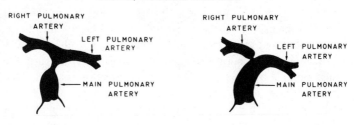

TYPE II
BIFURCATION STENOSIS

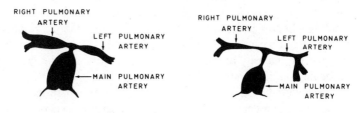

TYPE III
MULTIPLE, PERIPHERAL STENOSIS

TYPE IV
CENTRAL+PERIPHERAL STENOSIS

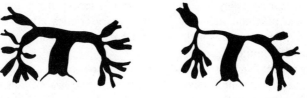

FIG 6–8.
Classification of peripheral pulmonary artery stenosis. (Modified from Gay BB Jr, et al: *AJR* 1963; 90:599.)

murmur. The chest roentgenogram will show right ventricular enlargement, a dilated main pulmonary artery, and normal vascular markings. The ECG will show right ventricular hypertrophy.

DIFFERENTIAL DIAGNOSIS

The patient with obstruction to right ventricular outflow must be differentiated from a patient with an atrial septal defect, a patent ductus arteriosus, and an innocent murmur.

The patient with an atrial septal defect will have a murmur, ejection in quality, and systolic in time at the same location, but it will be softer in intensity and will have a widely split second sound that does not vary with respiration.

The patient with a patent ductus arteriosus can be confused with one having pulmonary stenosis only if the diastolic portion of the murmur is not present consistently. If that is the case, echocardiography or cardiac catheterization may be necessary to effect the differential.

The patient with an innocent murmur has a softer murmur, a perfectly normal second sound, a normal chest roentgenogram, and a normal ECG.

PEARLS

1. Think "right ventricular outflow tract obstruction" when considering pulmonary stenosis, because it will instinctively urge you to consider all of the sites of potential obstruction.
2. Valvular pulmonary stenosis is more common in males than in females.
3. Pulmonary artery stenosis is seen frequently with rubella syndrome. These patients will not be well developed and well nourished.
4. Mild valvular pulmonary stenosis may be difficult to distinguish from an innocent murmur.
5. There is good correlation between the degree of stenosis and the degree of right ventricular hypertrophy on the ECG.
6. Malignant pulmonary stenosis is an extreme emergency and re-

quires the utmost speed in establishing a precise diagnosis. Until pulmonary flow is established, the patient is at risk of death from hypoxia.

7. If the diagnosis of pulmonary stenosis is suspected in a newborn, an echocardiogram can uncover an unrecognized ventricular septal defect, permitting a diagnosis of tetralogy of Fallot.

7

Coarctation of the Aorta

EMBRYOLOGY

Between the fifth and seventh weeks of gestation, the aortic arch develops. This begins as six paired arches proliferating from the distal end of the truncus arteriosus. While the right fourth arch participates in the development of the right subclavian artery, the left fourth arch becomes the definitive aortic arch connecting with the left dorsal aorta to complete the entire aorta (Fig 7–1).

ANATOMY

For reasons that are not known, the area of the aorta near the insertion of the ductus arteriosus may develop improperly, leaving a restricted lumen. This can take place proximal to, at, or distal to the insertion of the ductus arteriosus (Fig 7–2). It is on this basis that a classification of preductal or postductal coarctation of the aorta has been established. The entire aorta from the aortic valve into the abdominal aorta can be affected, but only the most common site in the vicinity of the ductus is considered. The precise location of the co-

85

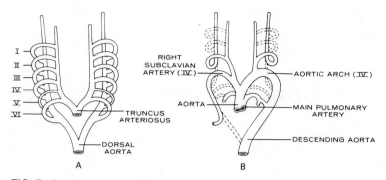

FIG 7–1.
Diagrammatic representation of the formation of the aortic arch. **A,** the primitive six arches originating from the distal end of the truncus arteriosus. **B,** the definitive form of the aorta, indicating its origin in the fourth arch.

arctation will affect the entire clinical picture; therefore, each is discussed individually.

PREDUCTAL COARCTATION OF THE AORTA

Hemodynamics

The coarctation obstructs flow from the proximal portion of the aorta to its distal portion. If the coarctation is proximal to the insertion of the ductus arteriosus, the lower half of the body will be supplied by the right ventricle through the ductus. The upper half of the body will be supplied by the left ventricle, and collateral circulation will not be stimulated during fetal life. After birth, the circuitry persists and can be conceptualized in the mnemonic

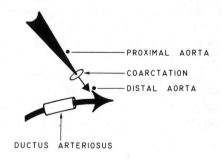

The arrows represent blood entering the descending aorta from the right ventricle through the ductus (heavy arrow) and to a much lesser degree from the ascending aorta (thin arrow). If the flow is followed with the relative size of the arrows kept in mind, the effect on the heart can be demonstrated by the following diagram:

RIGHT ATRIUM →	LEFT ATRIUM → ↑
RIGHT VENTRICLE ↑	LEFT VENTRICLE → ↑
MAIN PULMONARY ARTERY ↑	ASCENDING AORTA →
PULMONARY VESSELS →	DESCENDING AORTA ↑

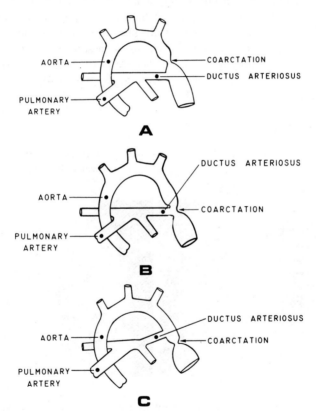

FIG 7–2.
Diagrammatic representation of the anatomical variations of coarctation of the aorta as it relates to the location of the ductus arteriosus. **A,** preductal; **B,** at the ductus; **C,** postductal.

The arrows represent alteration in the size of a vessel or a chamber as follows:

$\rightarrow$ Unchanged
$\uparrow$ Increased

Translated to the chest roentgenogram, one might expect a normal right atrium, enlarged right ventricle, a full pulmonary artery segment, and a prominent descending aorta. The left atrium and the left ventricle usually are unimpressive in size. The arch of the aorta might be diminished in size, but this usually is not apparent on the roentgenogram. Parenthetically, since this variation almost always appears in the newborn period, and since specific chamber enlargement is quite difficult to recognize in this age range, the usual chest roentgenogram may show only cardiomegaly (Fig 7–3). The electrocardiogram (ECG) will consistently show right ventricular hypertrophy (Fig 7–4).

Clinical Application

The patient—usually an infant—with preductal coarctation of the aorta should have differential cyanosis. The lower half of the body is

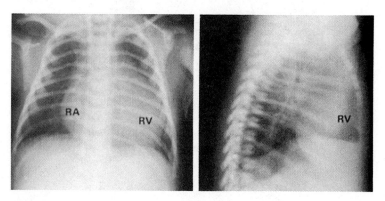

FIG 7–3.
Chest roentgenograms of a newborn with preductal coarctation of the aorta. Although the right atrium and the right ventricle are labeled, it would be more accurate to state that generalized cardiomegaly is present with normal pulmonary vascularity. *RA* = right atrium; *RV* = right ventricle.

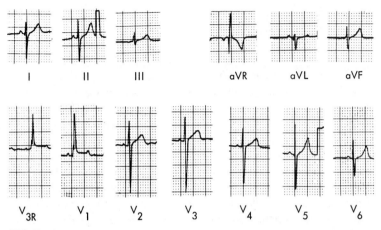

FIG 7–4.

Electrocardiogram of an infant with preductal coarctation of the aorta. The salient features are the dominant S_1 and R/S_{aVF}—right axis deviation. Also present are a dominant R wave in V_1 and S wave in $V_{5, 6}$, interpretable as right ventricular hypertrophy. The T wave in V_1 is also upright.

being supplied by the right ventricle and should be cyanotic, whereas the upper half of the body is being supplied by the left ventricle and should be totally oxygenated.

Theoretically, this is the case and can be demonstrated by obtaining simultaneous arterial blood samples for oxygen determination from the right radial artery and descending aorta. However, visually this occurs only rarely. (This is a common examination question.) Hypertension in the upper extremities and a lower pressure in the lower extremities can be expected. Because the right ventricle has been perfusing the lower half of the body throughout fetal life and continues to do so after birth, the femoral pulses will be present but diminished in amplitude and their onset will be delayed when compared to the radial pulse. Normally, no murmur is present. This is because collateral vessels normally are not present in any significant degree, and there is very little antegrade flow through the coarcted segment. A bicuspid aortic valve is a frequent coexisting lesion. If it is stenotic, its presence may be recognized by an ejection systolic murmur heard at the fourth interspace to the left of the sternum, with some transmission to the second interspace to the right of the sternum. The second sound will be closely split, with an intensification of the pulmonary component. This event is related to the persistence of fetal pulmonary hypertension.

If the patient is in congestive heart failure with poor cardiac output, the classic relationship of pulses and blood pressure in the upper and lower extremities will be obscured. Therefore, it makes reexamination of the patient, when compensated, an absolute necessity.

Therefore, a newborn can be suspected of having preductal coarctation of the aorta if he or she gets into early difficulty with congestive heart failure, demonstrates cyanosis of the lower half of the body, has prominent radial pulses with hypertension in the upper extremities and diminished femoral pulses and blood pressure in the lower extremities, shows right ventricular hypertrophy on the ECG, and demonstrates cardiomegaly in the chest x-ray film. Echocardiography has the capability of demonstrating the coarctation of the aorta (see Fig 7–8). Color flow Doppler can add a dimension to the imaging by demon-

TABLE 7–1.

Idealized Cardiac Catheterization Data in a Newborn With Preductal Coarctation of the Aorta*

Site	Pressure (mm Hg) Normal	Patient	Oxygen Saturation (%) Normal	Patient
Superior vena cava			70	70
Inferior vena cava			74	74
Right atrium	a = 5 v = 3 m = 4		72	72
Right ventricle	60/2	60/2	72	72
Main pulmonary artery	60/40	60/40	72	72
Left atrium	a = 5 v = 7 m = 6	a = 5 v = 7 m = 6	97	97
Left ventricle	60/5	90/5	97	97
Ascending aorta	60/40	90/40	97	97
Descending aorta	60/40	60/40	97	80

*The salient features are elevated pressures in the right ventricle and the main pulmonary artery. The pressure in the left ventricle and the ascending aorta is even higher. The pressure in the descending aorta is diminished. The oxygen saturation in the descending aorta is diminished.

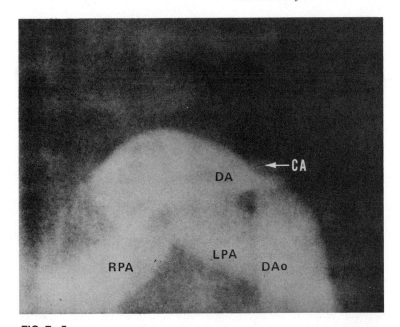

FIG 7–5.
An enlargement of a single frame of a 35-mm cineangiocardiogram performed in a newborn with preductal coarctation of the aorta. Note the insertion of the ductus arteriosus into the descending aorta distal to the site of the coarctation. *DA* = ductus arteriosus; *CA* = coarctation of the aorta; *DAo* = descending aorta; *RPA* = right pulmonary artery; *LPA* = left pulmonary artery.

strating the right-to-left shunt into the aorta below the site of the co-arctation (not demonstrated). If in doubt, the diagnosis can be proved with cardiac catheterization, during which the desaturation in the descending aorta and the relative hypertension in the ascending aorta will be shown (Table 7–1). Angiocardiography will clarify the pathologic findings (Fig 7–5).

POSTDUCTAL COARCTATION OF THE AORTA

Hemodynamics

The coarctation obstructs flow from the proximal portion of the aorta to its distal portion. With the coarctation being distal to the insertion of the ductus arteriosus, right ventricular flow will have been into the ascending aorta throughout all of fetal life. The presence of the coarctation would require the development of collateral circulation during fetal life to permit perfusion of the lower half of the body. This is indeed the case and is demonstrated in the mnemonic

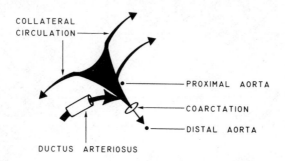

The heavy arrow represents blood flowing through the ductus into the proximal aorta. The coarctation restricts antegrade flow, as shown by the thin arrow in the distal aorta, and stimulates proximal flow, as shown by the multiple arrows in the collateral circulation. In the older infant or young child, the ductus normally closes and the fetal pulmonary hypertension resolves. If these facts are remembered and if the flow of blood now is followed with the mnemonic in mind, the effect on the heart and vessels can be demonstrated by the following diagram:

RIGHT ATRIUM →	LEFT ATRIUM → ↑
RIGHT VENTRICLE →	LEFT VENTRICLE ↑
MAIN PULMONARY ARTERY →	ASCENDING AORTA → ↑
PULMONARY VESSELS →	DESCENDING AORTA ↑

The arrows represent alteration in the size of a chamber or a vessel as follows:

→ Unchanged
↑ Increased

Translated to the chest roentgenogram, one would expect the right side of the heart to be normal, some possible enlargement of the left atrium, an enlarged left ventricle, and a dilated ascending aorta. The descending aorta would also show poststenotic dilatation, and on occasion, that relationship will be visible on the chest roentgenogram, resembling a figure "3" (Fig 7–6). The ECG would demonstrate varying degrees of left ventricular hypertrophy (Fig 7–7).

However, even in the presence of left ventricular hypertrophy (much as in aortic stenosis), the ECG may fail to show it and will be interpreted as normal.

Clinical Application

These patients' coloring is uniformly pink. Pulses in the upper extremities are full, whereas those in the lower extremities are diminished to absent. The blood pressure in the arms is elevated, whereas that in the legs is diminished. If the orifice of the coarctation is sufficient to permit flow through it, an ejection murmur occurring after the first sound and in the middle of systole may well be heard along the upper left paravertebral area. A bruit will be heard representing collateral flow through the dilated intercostal arteries throughout the entire

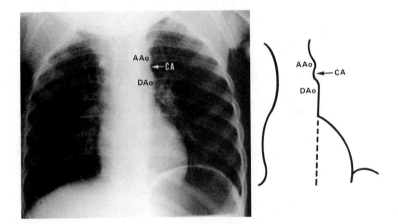

FIG 7–6.
Chest roentgenogram of a child with a postductal coarctation of the aorta. Note the indentation of the aorta resembling a figure "3." This is demonstrated in line form in the righthand panel. *AAo* = ascending aorta; *CA* = coarctation of the aorta; *DAo* = descending aorta.

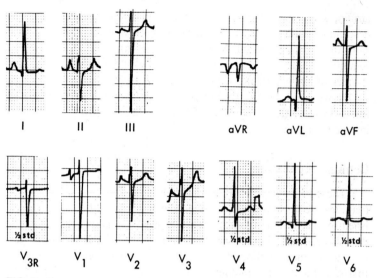

FIG 7–7.
Electrocardiogram of a child with postductal coarctation of the aorta. The salient features are a dominant R_1 and S_{aVF}—left axis deviation. Also present are a deep S wave in lead V_1 and a very tall R wave in leads $V_{5, 6}$, interpretable as left ventricular hypertrophy.

posterior aspect of the chest and through the dilated internal mammary arteries throughout the anterior aspect of the chest. If a bicuspid aortic valve is coexistent and stenotic, a harsh grade I-II/VI ejection systolic murmur will be heard at the second interspace to the right of the sternum, transmitting into the neck vessels. This murmur may be preceded by a systolic ejection click heard at the fourth interspace to the left of the sternum. It should be remembered that the click is heard over the site of the aortic valve itself and that the murmur is a transmitted sound of turbulent blood flow in the ascending aorta after it has passed the stenotic valve. Should the bicuspid valve be insufficient, a high-pitched decrescendo early to mid-diastolic murmur will be heard at the left third and fourth interspaces. The second sound generally is normal, with variable splitting and normal components. If the pressure in the ascending aorta is very high, the aortic component of the second sound should be increased in absolute intensity.

The infant with a postductal coarctation of the aorta follows one of two courses. Within the first 3 months of life, the infant may have congestive heart failure with the usual symptoms of cough and signs of tachypnea, dyspnea, tachycardia, and hepatosplenomegaly. At this time, the classic findings of full pulses and hypertension in the upper extremities and diminished pulses and blood pressure in the lower extremities may be obscured because of poor cardiac output. After the compensation, the classic findings will be more apparent, and, therefore, reexamination is mandatory.

The suprasternal long-axis view of the two-dimensional echocardiogram can provide an image of the arch of the aorta, the brachial cephalic vessels, and the site of the coarctation (Fig 7–8). In addition to clarifying the basic diagnosis, the echocardiogram with Doppler can further uncover coexisting lesions such as a ventricular septal defect and the previously mentioned bicuspid aortic valve, with or without stenosis. Should the echocardiogram not adequately clarify the clinical picture and the anatomy, cardiac catheterization can be performed. If catheterization is done, the difference in pressures in the ascending

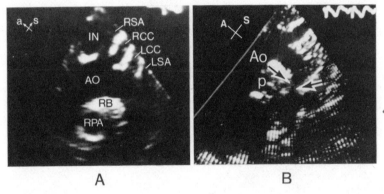

FIG 7–8.
Suprasternal long-axis view of an echocardiogram in a normal patient **(A)** and in a patient with coarctation of the aorta **(B)**. Note *arrows* in **B** pointing to a constriction in the descending aorta. A = anterior; S = superior; AO = aorta; RSA = right subclavian artery; RCC = right common carotid artery; LCC = left common carotid artery; LSA = left subclavian artery; RB = right bronchus; RPA and p = right pulmonary artery; IN = innominate vein. (From Silverman NH, Snider AR: *Two-Dimensional Echocardiography in Congenital Heart Disease.* Norwalk, Conn, Appleton-Century-Crofts, 1982, p 110. Used by permission.)

and descending aorta will be demonstrated (Table 7–2). At the same time it will permit clarification of any coexisting lesions.

Angiocardiography will demonstrate the pathologic characteristics (Fig 7–9). The majority of patients, however, accommodate to the coarctation and grow without trouble. The diagnosis can be established on the basis of the physical examination, with lesser support from the chest roentgenogram and the ECG. The exact site of the coarctation in the thoracic aorta can, in fact, be suspected on the basis of palpation alone. If a pulse is palpable in the right arm and absent in the left arm and legs, the coarctation is either proximal to or at the site of the left subclavian artery. If a pulse is palpable in the left arm and absent in the right arm and legs, the coarctation is distal to the left subclavian artery, but there is an anomalous right subclavian artery originating distal to the site of the coarctation. The presence of pulses in the right arm and right carotid but the absence of pulses in the left carotid, left arm, and legs suggests that the coarctation is at the isthmus.

TABLE 7–2.

Idealized Cardiac Catheterization Data in a Child With Postductal Coarctation of the Aorta*

Site	Pressure (mm Hg)		Oxygen Saturation (%)	
	Normal	Patient	Normal	Patient
Superior vena cava			70	70
Inferior vena cava			74	74
Right atrium	a = 5 v = 3 m = 4	a = 5 v = 3 m = 4	72	72
Right ventricle	25/2	25/2	72	72
Main pulmonary artery	25/12	25/12	72	72
Left atrium	a = 5 v = 7 m = 6	a = 5 v = 7 m = 6	97	97
Left ventricle	110/5	160/5	97	97
Ascending aorta	110/70	160/70	97	97
Descending aorta	110/70	70/50	97	97

*The salient feature is the presence of elevated pressures in the left ventricle and the ascending aorta with diminished pressures in the descending aorta. The oxygen saturations are entirely normal.

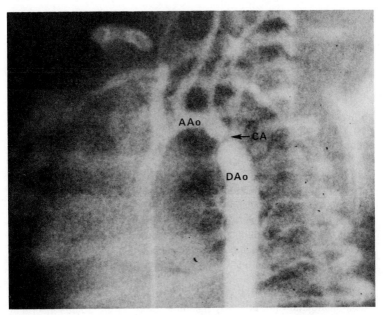

FIG 7–9.
Enlargement of a single frame of a 35-mm cineangiocardiogram performed in a child with postductal coarctation of the aorta. Note the site of the coarctation. No ductus is seen because it has closed spontaneously. *AAo* = ascending aorta; *CA* = coarctation of the aorta; *DAo* = descending aorta.

DIFFERENTIAL DIAGNOSIS

The lesion is not confused with many others. It must be differentiated from other noncardiac causes of hypertension, such as essential hypertension, renal pathologic conditions, and pheochromocytoma.

PEARLS

1. Coarctation of the aorta is more common in males than in females.
2. Coarctation can occur at any site in the aorta, and abdominal location should be looked for routinely.

3. Rib notching, a common finding in the older patient with coarctation of the aorta, normally does not occur before 8 years of age. It is a function of physical erosion of the undersurface of the ribs as a result of intercostal collateral circulation.

4. Bicuspid aortic valve occurs in approximately 50% of patients as a coexisting lesion.

5. Coarctation of the aorta is the most common cardiac abnormality in patients with Turner's syndrome.

6. In the first few days of life, the expected relationship of hypertension in the upper extremities and lower pressures in the legs in a preductal coarctation may be absent. A high index of suspicion is therefore warranted in the newborn with congestive heart failure.

7. Obtaining a valid reading of hypertension requires the choice of a proper-sized blood pressure cuff and the application of the occluding bladder appropriately over the brachial artery. (This is a very basic maneuver that is performed incorrectly with surprising frequency.) This caveat holds whether the blood pressure is obtained by traditional manometer method, flush technique, Doppler, or Dynamap.

8. A ventricular septal defect is frequently seen with a preductal coarctation of the aorta. The principles elucidated in the section on postductal coarctation are precisely the same as when the ductus inserts at the coarctation.

9. In the newborn, the presence of a patent ductus arteriosus may confound the physical examination and make the diagnosis more difficult.

PART III

Right-to-Left Shunts

8

Differential Diagnosis of Cyanotic Heart Disease

One of the challenges a physician who cares for children faces is a patient, generally a newborn, who appears "dusky," the general descriptive term applied to cyanosis. The differential diagnosis of such a patient falls into the familiar and well-known "five Ts." With some license taken with the letter T, these are tetralogy of Fallot and its extreme variation, pulmonary atresia with ventricular septal defect; tricuspid atresia; and a subset of pulmonary atresia with intact ventricular septum, transposition of the great arteries, truncus arteriosus, and total anomalous pulmonary venous connection. Also in the differential, but not relating to the letter T and much less common, would be lesions such as Ebstein's anomaly, malposition of the heart with mixed complex intracardiac pathology, single ventricle with mixed complex intracardiac pathology, double outlet right ventricle, and double inlet left ventricle. This chapter deals with the basic five Ts and their subsets, because they make up far and away the most likely ultimate diagnosis.

It is axiomatic, but it must be said that when a nurse reports the presence of duskiness in a newborn, an evaluation is essential. That evaluation must include a review of the prenatal and perinatal events

TABLE 8–1.
A Guideline to the Differential Diagnosis of a Patient With Cyanotic Heart Disease

Lesion	Salient Findings on Physical Examination	ECG Interpretation	Radiographic Findings	Refer to Chapter
A. Tetralogy of Fallot, classic	1. Systolic ejection murmur second left interspace transmitted to the back 2. Second sound single 3. Cyanosis mild or nonexistent in the newborn 4. In no acute distress	1. Right ventricular hypertrophy 2. Right-axis deviation	1. Normal-sized heart, elevated apex, right ventricular enlargement (boot-shaped heart) 2. Decreased vascularity 3. Right aortic arch 4. May be perfectly normal	9
A₁. Pulmonary atresia with ventricular septal defect. (Conceptual variation of tetralogy of Fallot)	1. Inconsistent systolic ejection murmur or no murmur at all 2. Second sound single 3. Cyanosis easily apparent and severe 4. Comfortable until patent ductus arteriosus begins to close, then dyspneic	1. Right ventricular hypertrophy 2. Right-axis deviation	1. Normal-sized heart, elevated apex, right ventricular enlargement 2. Decreased vascularity	9
B. Tricuspid atresia	1. Variable murmurs or none at all 2. Second sound single 3. Cyanosis tends to be severe 4. Comfort varies	1. Left ventricular hypertrophy 2. Left-axis deviation (0 to −90 degrees)	1. Generally normal-sized heart with elevated apex (all left ventricular enlargement with posterior displacement on lateral view) 2. Decreased vascularity	10

B₁. Pulmonary atresia with intact ventricular septum	1. Usually no murmur 2. Second sound single 3. Cyanosis tends to be severe 4. Comfortable until patent ductus arteriosus begins to close	1. Left ventricular hypertrophy 2. Normal (0–90 degrees) or right axis (90–180 degrees) deviation	1. Generally normal-sized heart with elevated apex (all left ventricular enlargement with posterior displacement on lateral view) 2. Decreased vascularity	10
C. Transposition of the great arteries with intact ventricular septum	1. Usually no murmur 2. Second sound single 3. Cyanosis visibly mild and may be missed 4. Comfortable until patent ductus arteriosus begins to close	1. Right ventricular hypertrophy 2. May be normal	1. Generalized cardiomegaly 2. Narrow mediastinum 3. Increased vascularity 4. May be normal	11
D₁. Truncus arteriosus Types I, II, and III	1. Systolic ejection murmur at the second left interspace or continuous murmur at the second left interspace or no murmur 2. Second sound single 3. Cyanosis visibly mild	1. Combined ventricular hypertrophy	1. Cardiomegaly 2. Increased vascularity (the main, right, and left pulmonary arteries may be particularly prominent in a more cranial position than than usually seen)	12

(Continued.)

TABLE 8–1 (cont.).

Lesion	Salient Findings on Physical Examination	ECG Interpretation	Radiographic Findings	Refer to Chapter
(Continued.)				
D₂: Type IV	1. Systolic ejection murmur or continuous murmurs on the anterior or posterior side of the chest 2. Second sound single 3. Cyanosis severe	1. Right ventricular hypertrophy	1. Mild cardiomegaly with elevated apex (boot-shaped heart) 2. Decreased vascularity	12
E. Total anomalous pulmonary venous connection with obstruction	1. Little or no murmur 2. Second sound may be duplicated 3. Dyspneic, tachypneic, and possibly rales 4. Possible hepatomegaly 5. In marked respiratory distress 6. Cyanosis varies and may be mild	1. Right ventricular hypertrophy	1. Small cardiac size 2. Pulmonary venous congestion, pulmonary edema	13

and a physical examination. Not all patients with cyanosis necessarily have congenital heart disease as the etiology. The differential diagnosis of cyanosis must also include polycythemia of the newborn caused by fetal-fetal or maternal-fetal transfusion, pulmonary problems such as atelectasis, hypoplasia, lobar emphysema, or other less common congenital malformations, neurologic abnormalities resulting in depression of respirations, metabolic disturbances, hypoglycemia, and sepsis.

Laboratory studies would then be necessary to help clarify the problem. Included would be a complete blood cell count, chest roentgenogram, electrocardiogram (ECG), and an arterial blood gas drawn in room air and in an atmosphere of high concentration of oxygen.

The details of the events surrounding the delivery plus the physical examination would help eliminate the neurologic system as the etiology. The blood count would rule out polycythemia of the newborn. The chest roentgenogram would assist in evaluating the cardiovascular system, but equally so, the lungs. The arterial blood gas used with the concept of the hyperoxic test will assist in determining that the patient likely has cyanotic congenital heart disease. An arterial blood gas at room air that has a partial pressure of oxygen (po_2) in the 25 to 30 mm Hg range in the presence of normal partial pressure of carbon dioxide (pco_2) and no acidosis will not significantly increase when challenged with oxygen if the cause is cyanotic congenital heart disease. If, however, the depressed po_2 value is caused by inadequate pulmonary function, one would expect to see an increase in the po_2 value of at least 100 mm Hg over the baseline number.

If the basic work-up and laboratory studies direct you to the probability of cyanotic congenital heart disease, Table 8–1 will assist in your differential diagnosis and direct you to a specific chapter in the book for details.

PEARLS

1. A low po_2 value drawn within the first 1 or 2 hours of life may be misleading and needs to be rechecked as an infant gets several hours older.

2. Do not be misled if a po_2 value of 35 mm Hg increases to 95 or

even 105 mm Hg with oxygen, because a lesion such as truncus arteriosus can do that.

3. A finesse: If you are involved with an absolute emergency and cannot see the patient immediately, having an arterial blood gas performed with and without oxygen will give you powerful information before the physical examination and review of the history and at the same time will permit you to handle the emergency.

4. Be reminded that a measurement of oxygen saturation with a pulse oximeter is not a substitute for an arterial blood sample when applying the hyperoxic test (it is not even a substitute for an adequate physical examination and the thought process).

9 | Tetralogy of Fallot

EMBRYOLOGY

Toward the end of the third week and into the fourth, the common trunk normally is divided into the pulmonary artery and the aorta. This is accomplished by the development of the truncoconal ridges, which grow caudad in a spiral fashion, resulting in the posterior lateral origin of the aorta and the anterior medial origin of the pulmonary artery (Fig 9–1). This septum fuses with the bulbar ridges, which, in turn, participate with the endocardial cushions and membranous proliferation from the ventricular septum to form the definitive closure of the interventricular septum (Fig 9–2).

Between the fourth and eighth weeks of gestation, the single ventricular chamber is effectively divided into two. This is accomplished by fusion of the membranous portion of the ventricular septum, the endocardial cushions, and the bulbus cordis (the proximal portion of the truncus arteriosus). The muscular portion of the ventricular septum grows cephalad as each ventricular chamber enlarges, eventually meeting with the right and left ridges of the bulbus cordis. The right ridge fuses with the tricuspid valve and the endocardial cushion, thus sepa-

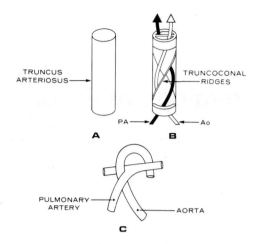

FIG 9–1.
Diagrammatic representation of the division of the truncus arteriosus **(A)** into the aorta and pulmonary artery **(C)**. **B** shows the septation and the spiral direction of the pulmonary artery and the aorta. *PA* = pulmonary artery; *Ao* = aorta.

rating the pulmonary valve from the tricuspid valve. The left ridge fuses with a ridge of the interventricular septum, leaving the aortic ring in continuity with the mitral ring. The endocardial cushions are concomitantly developing and ultimately fuse with the bulbar ridges and the muscular portion of the septum. The final closure and separation of the two ventricles is made by the fibrous tissue of the membranous portion of the interventricular septum (Fig 9–3).

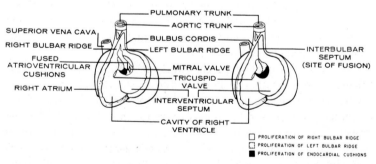

FIG 9–2.
Schematic representation of the role of the bulbus cordis in the formation of the interventricular septum. (See text for explanation.)

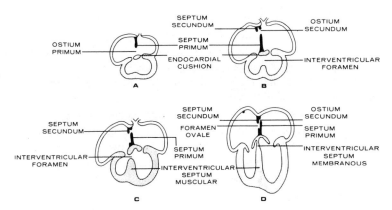

FIG 9–3.
Schematic representation of the formation of the interventricular septum. **A,** 30 days; **B,** 33 days; **C,** 37 days; **D,** newborn. (See text for explanation.) (Modified from Moss AJ, Adams FH [eds]: *Heart Disease in Infants, Children and Adolescents.* Baltimore, Williams & Wilkins Co, 1968, p 16.)

ANATOMY

Essentially two theories are proposed in an attempt to explain the tetralogy of Fallot. The first relates merely to an abnormality in the septation of the truncus. It is postulated that if this septation is asymmetric, the two great vessels will be of unequal size. Because of the asymmetry, that portion of the septum that participates in closure of the atrioventricular area will not be available, and a ventricular septal defect will result. The asymmetry will also lead to a greater than normal amount of tissue in the infundibulum of the right ventricle, which then would account for the infundibular stenosis. The other theory relates the entire clinical picture to an abnormality in development of the infundibular area of the right ventricle. It is believed that the infundibular stenosis restricts blood flow through the pulmonary artery during fetal life, causing it to be smaller than normal at the time of birth. Increased blood flow through the aorta during fetal life causes it to be large at the time of birth. The improper development of the infundibular area also disturbs the normal completion of the atrioventricular canal, and a resultant ventricular septal defect occurs.

Whichever theory is accepted, a consistent hypertrophy of the crista supraventricularis, a frequent hypoplasia of the pulmonary valve anulus with stenosis of the pulmonary valves themselves, and a ventricular septal defect located below the crista supraventricularis generally approximating the size of the aorta result. The crista supraventricularis, by definition, is a muscular ridge located below the pulmonary valves, separating the infundibulum from the remainder of the right ventricular cavity (Fig 9–4).

Traditionally, tetralogy of Fallot has been defined as consisting of four basic anatomical abnormalities: infundibular stenosis, ventricular septal defect, right ventricular hypertrophy, and overriding or dextroposition of the aorta. From an anatomical standpoint, this remains the case, but from a physiologic standpoint, I believe that only the in-

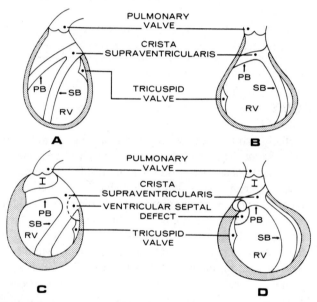

FIG 9–4.

Diagrammatic representation of the appearance of the crista supraventricularis and its parietal and septal bands in a normal patient and in a patient with tetralogy of Fallot. **A,** normal—lateral view; **B,** normal—anteroposterior view; **C,** tetralogy of Fallot—lateral view; **D,** tetralogy of Fallot—anteroposterior view. Note the increased size in the parietal band and septal band and the presence of a ventricular septal defect in **C** and **D**. *PB* = parietal band; *SB* = septal band; *RV* = right ventricle; *I* = infundibulum.

fundibular stenosis and the ventricular septal defect are of importance. The right ventricular hypertrophy is secondary to the obstruction to right ventricular ejection, and the aorta receives poorly oxygenated blood because of the obstruction of right ventricular ejection in the presence of a ventricular septal defect without regard to the degree of physical overriding of the aorta.

If the physiologic parameters are accepted for the criteria of diagnosis, one patient may have very mild infundibular stenosis, be minimally cyanotic, and be considered as having a "pink tetralogy," whereas another would have obliteration of the outflow tract, be exceptionally cyanotic, and be considered as having pulmonary atresia. In fact, such a panorama exists. I have chosen, however, to use the remainder of the chapter to deal with what might loosely be called "classic tetralogy of Fallot," in which infundibular stenosis, a ventricular septal defect approximating the size of the aorta, and right ventricular pressures that are systemic in height are present. Hypoplasia of the pulmonary valve anulus and stenosis of the valves are present so commonly as to be considered virtually an integral part of the pathologic complex.

HEMODYNAMICS

The patient with tetralogy of Fallot has diminished blood flow to the lungs and increased blood flow to the body. This is demonstrated in the mnemonic

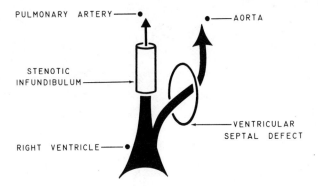

The small arrow entering the pulmonary artery represents diminished blood flow through the stenotic infundibulum. The heavier arrow represents flow of venous blood through the ventricular septal defect into the aorta. The thick black area identified as the right ventricle indicates the increased pressure in that chamber. If the blood flow is followed with mnemonic in mind, the effect on the heart can be demonstrated by the following diagram:

RIGHT ATRIUM → ↑   LEFT ATRIUM →
RIGHT VENTRICLE ↑   LEFT VENTRICLE →
MAIN PULMONARY ARTERY ↓   AORTA ↑
PULMONARY VESSELS ↓

The arrows represent alteration in the size of a chamber or a vessel as follows:

→ Unchanged
↑ Increased
↓ Decreased

This information can be translated to the chest roentgenogram, where one would expect to see possible enlargement of the right

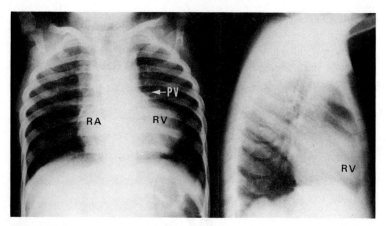

FIG 9–5.
Chest roentgenograms of a patient with tetralogy of Fallot. Note the enlarged right atrium and right ventricle and decreased pulmonary vessels. The overall appearance is that of a boot-shaped heart. *RA* = right atrium; *RV* = right ventricle; *PV* = pulmonary vessels.

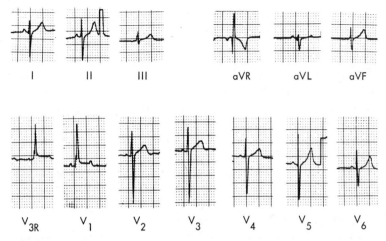

FIG 9–6.
Electrocardiogram of a patient with tetralogy of Fallot. The salient features are the dominant S_1 and R/S_{aVF}— right axis deviation. Also present are a dominant R wave in V_1 and an S wave in $V_{5,6}$, interpretable as right ventricular hypertrophy. The T wave in V_1 is also upright.

atrium, definite enlargement of the right ventricle, a small main pulmonary artery, and a normal left atrium and left ventricle—recognized as a boot-shaped heart. The aorta would be enlarged. In 25% of patients, the aorta arches to the right (Fig 9–5). The electrocardiogram (ECG) would show right ventricular hypertrophy (Fig 9–6).

CLINICAL APPLICATION

Many believe that the infundibular hypertrophy intrinsic to tetralogy of Fallot increases progressively with age and, as such, increases the right-to-left shunting through the ventricular septal defect. If this is the case, it can offer an explanation for the delayed appearance of cyanosis. With time and persistent cyanosis, the fingers and toes become clubbed, and squatting occurs. As right ventricular hypertrophy progresses, the ventricle encroaches on the retrosternal space, and its contractions can be felt as a heave along the left sternal border. The first sound will be normal. Generally, no ejection click will be heard. The aorta, because of its malposition, is closer to the chest wall than usual, and its valve closure is heard more easily. The infundibular stenosis is responsible for a prolonged ejection time of the right ventricle, which greatly delays the closing of the pulmonary valve. The valve itself frequently is thickened and is relatively immobile, causing it to close with decreased intensity. This all results in a single second sound to auscultation, which can be recorded as a very widely duplicated event with marked diminution of the pulmonary component. The murmur, related to flow through the infundibulum, will be heard in the second and third interspaces to the left of the sternum, be systolic in time, ejection in quality, and transmitted into the pulmonary vessels.

As a result of the restricted blood flow, collateral circulation through bronchial vessels or other aortic pulmonary communications develops occasionally. Its presence will be recognized as continuous murmurs, generally heard over the back.

The cyanosis is responsible for a number of secondary events. The relative hypoxemia tends to stimulate red blood cell production. If oral intake of iron is insufficient for the increased number of red blood cells, an iron-deficiency anemia will result. This diagnosis may be elusive because the patient may have a normal hemoglobin level for his or her age but still have a relative anemia. Therefore, a hematocrit reading and red blood cell indices must also be obtained to ensure an accurate hematologic evaluation. The polycythemia so commonly present increases the risk of development of a cerebral thrombosis and hemiplegia. Transient cerebral ischemia can occur, leading to paleness, limpness, and unconsciousness—the spells of tetralogy of Fallot. The right-to-left shunting through the ventricular septal defect increases the risk for cerebral abscesses.

The diagnosis of tetralogy of Fallot can be suspected in a patient in whom cyanosis develops in the middle of the first year of life, who has a prominent left side of the chest with a right ventricular heave, a single second sound, a systolic ejection murmur at the second and third interspaces to the left of the sternum, a chest roentgenogram showing the classic boot-shaped heart with diminished pulmonary vascular markings, and an ECG showing right ventricular hypertrophy. No single view of the echocardiogram can make a diagnosis of tetralogy of Fallot. However, the parasternal long-axis view can demonstrate the enlarged overriding aorta (Fig 9–7), and the parasternal short-axis view can show the thickened pulmonary valve (Fig 9–8).

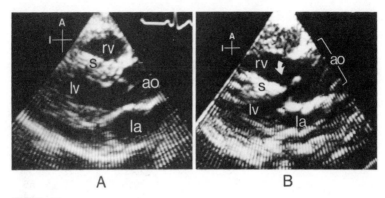

FIG 9–7.
Parasternal long-axis view of an echocardiogram in a normal patient **(A)** and a patient with tetralogy of Fallot **(B).** Note overriding of the ventricular septum by the aorta and presence of a ventricular septal defect (*white arrow* in **B** points to echo dropout in septum). A = anterior; *I* = inferior; *rv* = right ventricle, *s* = septum; *lv* = left ventricle; *la* = left atrium; *ao* = aorta. (From Silverman NH, Snider AR: *Two-Dimensional Echocardiography in Congenital Heart Disease.* Norwalk, Conn, Appleton-Century-Crofts, 1982. Used by permission.)

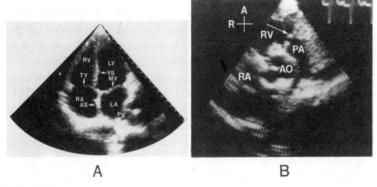

FIG 9–8.
Parasternal short-axis view of an echocardiogram in a normal patient **(A)** and in a patient with tetralogy of Fallot **(B).** Thin *white arrow* in **B** points to a thickened pulmonary valve. Also note the relatively small pulmonary artery *(PA).* A = anterior; R = right; *RV* = right ventricle; *TV* = tricuspid valve; *RA* = right atrium; *LA* = left atrium; *AO* = aorta. (From Silverman NH, Snider AR: *Two-Dimensional Echocardiography in Congenital Heart Disease.* Norwalk, Conn, Appleton-Century-Crofts, 1982, p 150. Used by permission.)

TABLE 9–1.

Idealized Cardiac Catheterization Data in a Child With Tetralogy of Fallot*

Site	Pressure (mm Hg)		Oxygen Saturation (%)	
	Normal	Patient	Normal	Patient
Superior vena cava			70	54
Inferior vena cava			74	60
Right atrium	a = 5 v = 3 m = 4	a = 9 v = 7 m = 6	72	55
Right ventricle				
Body	25/2	120/2	72	56
Infundibulum	25/2	70/2	72	56
Main pulmonary artery	25/2	20/10	72	56
Systemic artery	120/80	120/80	97	80

*The salient feature is generalized low oxygen saturations on the right side of the heart with desaturation in the systemic artery. There are systemic pressure in the body of the right ventricle, diminished pressure in the infundibulum, and very low pressure in the main pulmonary artery. There also is a slight elevation of the pressure in the right atrium.

The composite interpretation of the two views thus supports the diagnosis. Further confirmation, and more important, delineation of the specific pathologic characteristics, can be accomplished with cardiac catheterization. This will show systemic pressures in the right ventricle, diminished pressures in the infundibular area, markedly diminished pressure in the pulmonary artery, and arterial desaturation (Table 9–1). Cineangiocardiography would demonstrate the ventricular septal defect, infundibular stenosis, the displaced and enlarged aorta, and the degree of hypoplasia of the pulmonary arteries (Figs 9–9 and 9–10).

DIFFERENTIAL DIAGNOSIS

The patient with tetralogy of Fallot must be differentiated from one having severe valvular pulmonary stenosis with an intact ventricular septum, truncus arteriosus with diminished pulmonary flow (type IV), Eisenmenger's complex, origin of both great vessels from the

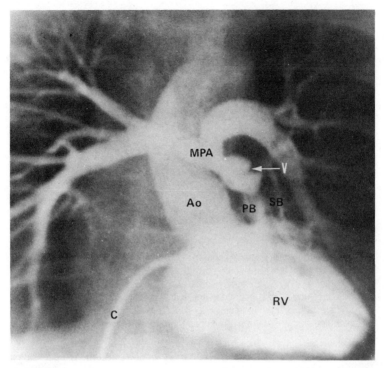

FIG 9–9.
Enlargement of a single frame from a cineangiocardiogram (anteroposterior projection) in a patient with tetralogy of Fallot. Note the narrow infundibulum bordered by the parietal band and septal band, the small pulmonary valve and main pulmonary artery, and the enlarged aorta, which is being filled from the right ventricle. *C* = catheter; *RV* = right ventricle; *PB* = parietal band; *SB* = septal band; *V* = pulmonary valve; *MPA* = main pulmonary artery; *Ao* = aorta.

right ventricle with pulmonary stenosis, transposition of the great arteries with subpulmonic stenosis and ventricular septal defect, and tricuspid atresia.

The patient with severe pulmonary stenosis—also called malignant pulmonary stenosis—is discussed in Chapter 6. Although he or she will have cyanosis at about the same age as the patient with tetralogy of Fallot, this patient will be severely ill with intense congestive heart failure and diminishing murmurs. Echocardiography generally

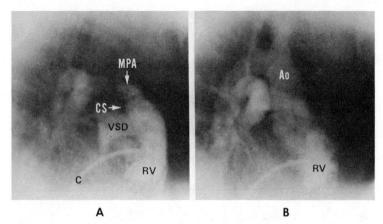

FIG 9–10.
Enlargement of two frames from a cineangiocardiogram (lateral projection) in a patient with tetralogy of Fallot. **A,** note the presence of the small main pulmonary artery arising from the right ventricle with the presence of the thickened crista supraventricularis. The ventricular septal defect is seen. **B,** taken several milliseconds later, note the presence of the aorta as it fills from the right ventricle. *C* = catheter; *RV* = right ventricle; *VSD* = ventricular septal defect; *CS* = crista supraventricularis; *MPA* = main pulmonary artery; *Ao* = aorta.

will identify the presence of an intact ventricular septum. If necessary, cardiac catheterization can be used.

On clinical grounds alone, the patient with truncus arteriosus may be quite difficult to distinguish from one having tetralogy of Fallot. Echocardiography and, if necessary, cardiac catheterization, will permit the differentiation.

The patient with Eisenmenger's complex may be momentarily confused with one having tetralogy of Fallot. The presence of cardiomegaly and increased vascular markings in the hilar area of the lungs, as seen on chest roentgenogram, will be useful in the differential diagnosis. Cardiac catheterization can finally delineate the two.

The patient with both great vessels arising from the right ventricle with pulmonary stenosis behaves physiologically quite like one with tetralogy of Fallot. However, basic to the lesion is separation of the normal continuity between the aortic ring and the mitral ring. This can be demonstrated on an echocardiogram or with a cineangiocardiogram.

The patient with transposition of the great arteries with ventricular septal defect and subpulmonic stenosis is discussed in detail in Chapter 11. He or she may be difficult to distinguish from one having tetralogy of Fallot, because both have an enlarged right ventricle, diminished pulmonary vascular markings, and a single second sound. The chest roentgenogram and the ECG are reminiscent of each other. However, echocardiography and, if necessary, cardiac catheterization will delineate the two.

The patient with tricuspid atresia will be of concern only on the basis of cyanosis but will be easily differentiated once an ECG is done. The presence of left ventricle hypertrophy will make the distinction.

PEARLS

1. This lesion occurs equally in males and females.

2. Congestive heart failure is extraordinarily rare, and its presence should direct your attention initially elsewhere.

3. An apparently normal hemoglobin level in a cyanotic patient should be evaluated further for iron-deficiency anemia.

4. A right aortic arch is seen in approximately 25% of the patients.

5. Rarely, the left pulmonary artery may be totally absent.

6. Remember that the murmur in tetralogy of Fallot is generated by flow through the stenotic infundibular area.

7. The patient with a "tet spell" has a marked decrease in the intensity of the murmur.

8. A "tet spell" can be confused with a seizure in the young infant. (Pay attention to the presence or absence of the previously recognized murmur.)

9. In 10% of patients with tetralogy of Fallot, the left anterior descending coronary artery arises from the right, rather than the left, coronary artery.

10

Tricuspid Atresia

EMBRYOLOGY

At about the fifth week of gestation there is a blending of the anterior endocardial cushion, the posterior endocardial cushion, a portion of the interventricular septum and the ventricular muscle itself to form the right atrioventricular valve, also known as the tricuspid valve (Figs 10–1 and 10–2).

The papillary muscles and the chordae tendineae arise from careful sculpturing of ventricular muscle (Fig 10–3).

ANATOMY

If there is a disruption between the balance of proliferation and resorption of tissue, the valve leaflets will not form normally. By definition, in tricuspid atresia no vestige of valvular tissue can be found and no communication between the right atrium and the right ventricle is possible. As in almost all types of congenital heart disease, subclas-

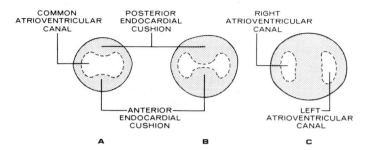

FIG 10–1.
Schematic representation of the common atrioventricular canal developing into a right and left canal. **A,** 30 days; **B,** 33 days; **C,** 35 days. (See text for explanation.) (Modified from Moss AJ, Adams FH [eds]: *Heart Disease in Infants, Children and Adolescents.* Baltimore, Williams & Wilkins Co, 1968, p 17.)

sifications exist. In tricuspid atresia, this classification depends on the relationship of the great vessels and the nature of the ventricular septum and pulmonary valve. A composite classification (Fig 10–4) from multiple sources is as follows:

I—*Normally related great vessels*
    a. No ventricular septal defect and pulmonary atresia
    b. Small ventricular septal defect and pulmonary stenosis

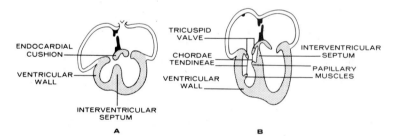

FIG 10–2.
Schematic representation of the formation of the tricuspid valve. (See text for explanation.) Identification of left-sided structures has been omitted intentionally. **A,** 37 days; **B,** newborn. (Modified from Moss AJ, Adams FH [eds]: *Heart Disease in Infants, Children and Adolescents.* Baltimore, Williams & Wilkins Co, 1968, p 16.)

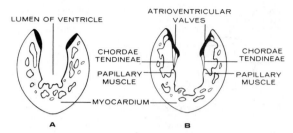

FIG 10–3.
Schematic representation of the formation of the atrioventricular valves and their chordae tendineae and papillary muscles. (See text for explanation.) **A** and **B**, progressive stages of development. (Modified from Moss AJ, Adams FH [eds]: *Heart Disease in Infants, Children and Adolescents.* Baltimore, Williams & Wilkins Co, 1968, p 19.)

    c. Large ventricular septal defect without pulmonary stenosis (not demonstrated)

II—*Transposition of the great arteries*
    a. Ventricular septal defect and pulmonary atresia
    b. Ventricular septal defect and pulmonary stenosis
    c. Ventricular septal defect without pulmonary stenosis (not demonstrated)

HEMODYNAMICS

Regardless of the intricacies implicit in the classification, the flow through the heart is essentially the same and is depicted in the mnemonic

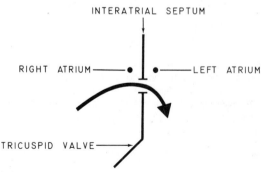

TRICUSPID ATRESIA WITHOUT TRANSPOSITION

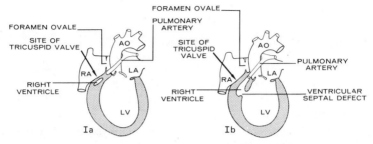

TRICUSPID ATRESIA WITH TRANSPOSITION

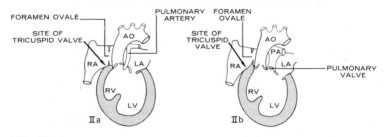

FIG 10–4.

Classification of tricuspid atresia. **Ia,** note the absence of a ventricular septal defect and the presence of pulmonary atresia. There is a rudimentary right ventricle. **Ib,** note the presence of a small ventricular septal defect and pulmonary stenosis. The right ventricle is small. **IIa,** note the presence of a large ventricular septal defect and pulmonary atresia. The right ventricle is fairly large. **IIb,** note the presence of a large ventricular septal defect and pulmonary stenosis with a relatively normal sized main pulmonary artery. RA = right atrium; LA = left atrium; LV = left ventricle; AO = aorta; and PA = pulmonary artery.

The arrow represents blood flowing from the right atrium through the interatrial septum and into the left atrium. If the blood flow is followed with this mnemonic in mind, the effect on the heart can be demonstrated by the following diagram:

RIGHT ATRIUM ↑	LEFT ATRIUM ↑
RIGHT VENTRICLE ↓	LEFT VENTRICLE ↑
PULMONARY ARTERY ↓	AORTA ↑
LUNGS ↓	

The arrows represent alteration in the size of a chamber or a vessel as follows:

↑ Increased
↓ Decreased

This information can logically be translated to the roentgenogram, where one would expect to find an enlarged right atrium, left atrium, left ventricle, and aorta. The vascular markings to the lungs would be diminished (Fig 10–5). The electrocardiogram (ECG) would also show right atrial, left atrial, and left ventricular hypertrophy. The axis will be leftward (Fig 10–6).

CLINICAL APPLICATION

The physical findings will rather clearly relate to the anatomy as described. The patient will be cyanotic and usually deeply so. The precordium will not be particularly prominent, but there may be a left ventricular thrust. The first sound will be single, its tricuspid portion

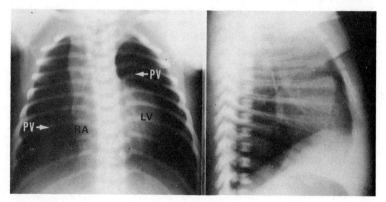

FIG 10–5.
Chest roentgenograms of a patient with tricuspid atresia. Note the cardiomegaly, elevated apex (but because of the left ventricular enlargement), and the prominent right atrium. The pulmonary markings are diminished. *LV* = left ventricle; *RA* = right atrium; *PV* = pulmonary vessels.

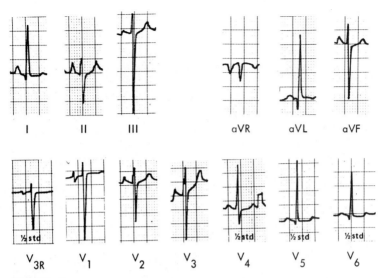

FIG 10-6.
Electrocardiogram of a patient with tricuspid atresia. The salient features are a tall P wave in II—right atrial hypertrophy. The deep S wave in V_1 and tall R waves in $V_{5,6}$ are interpretable as left ventricular hypertrophy. The negative P wave in V_{3R} suggests left atrial hypertrophy. The dominant R_1 and SaVF are left-axis deviation.

absent. The second sound usually will be single, but there may be a semblance of pulmonary component if there is a stenotic pulmonary valve (one of the rarer varieties). The nature of the murmur is variable at best. One might hear a diastolic murmur because of the flow across the mitral valve. If the ventricular septal defect is significant, a holo-systolic murmur may be present at the lower left sternal border. If pulmonary stenosis is present, an ejection murmur from flow through the stenotic valve can be anticipated. Last and most common, no murmur at all may be heard.

Characteristically, the patient with this lesion will become cyanotic in early infancy. Hypoxic spells are common, and right ventricular failure may occur also. The diagnosis can be suspected on the basis of the chest roentgenogram showing diminished vascular markings and the ECG showing left axis deviation and pure left ventricular hypertrophy. The two-dimensional echocardiogram in the apical four-chamber view is able to vividly demonstrate the pathology (Fig 10–7).

The details of the diagnosis can be elaborated on with cardiac catheterization, during which elevated pressures in both atria, inability to enter the right ventricle, and decreased saturation in the left atrium, left ventricle, and systemic artery will be found (Table 10–1). Clarification is obtained with angiocardiography, because the flow of dye goes from the right atrium to the left atrium, to the left ventricle, and out the aorta. A radiolucent area replaces the expected location of the right ventricle (Figs 10–8 and 10–9). Pulmonary blood flow is established through either a ductus arteriosus, bronchial circulation, or, when present, a small ventricular septal defect that leads to the pulmonary artery.

It should be mentioned that types Ic and IIc (see preceding classi-

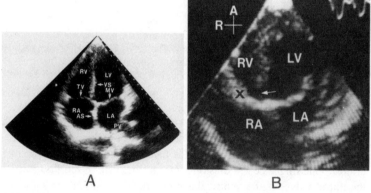

A   B

FIG 10–7.
Apical four-chamber view of an echocardiogram in a normal patient **(A)** and in a patient with tricuspid atresia **(B)**. Note in **B** the thickened echo density in the area of the tricuspid valve *(black X)* and the *white arrow* pointing to the echo-free space high in the ventricular septum. *A* = anterior; *R* = right; *RV* = right ventricle; *TV* = tricuspid valve; *RA* = right atrium; *LA* = left atrium; *MV* = tricuspid valve; *LV* = left ventricle; *LPV* = left pulmonary vein; *MB* = moderator band. (From Silverman NH, Snider AR: *Two-Dimensional Echocardiography in Congenital Heart Disease.* Norwalk, Conn, Appleton-Century-Crofts, 1982, p 195. Used by permission.)

TABLE 10–1.

Idealized Cardiac Catheterization Data in a Newborn With Tricuspid Atresia*

Site	Pressure (mm Hg)		Oxygen Saturation (%)	
	Normal	Patient	Normal	Patient
Superior vena cava			70	41
Inferior vena cava			74	45
Right atrium	a = 5 v = 3 m = 4	a = 12 v = 8 m = 7	72	45
Right ventricle	60/2	Not entered	72	Not entered
Main pulmonary artery	60/40	Not entered	72	Not entered
Left atrium	a = 5 v = 7 m = 6	a = 10 v = 8 m = 7	97	58
Left ventricle	60/5	60/5	97	58
Systemic artery	60/40	60/40	97	58
Pulmonary vein	a = 5 v = 7 m = 7	a = 10 v = 8 m = 8	97	97

*The salient features are elevated pressures in the right and left atria and failure to enter the right ventricle. There is a decrease in the oxygen saturation in the left atrium compared with the pulmonary veins (suggesting a right-to-left shunt across the atrial septum). Peripheral saturation is also diminished.

fication), each of which has a large ventricular septal defect without pulmonary stenosis, manifest in a different fashion. The increased pulmonary flow may result in left ventricular failure, and the clinical picture more closely resembles the findings in a patient with a ventricular septal defect but with mild cyanosis. The heart would be larger on roentgenogram and the vessels increased. The ECG would show more right ventricular hypertrophy than in the other types (not illustrated).

DIFFERENTIAL DIAGNOSIS

Initially, the patient with tricuspid atresia must be differentiated from one having transposition of the great arteries, truncus arteriosus,

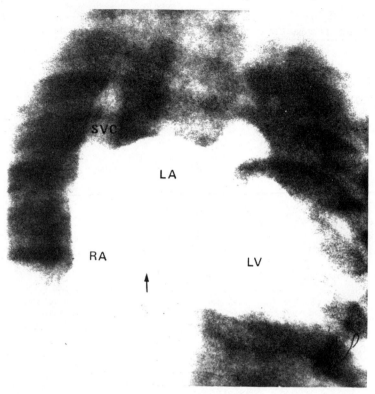

FIG 10–8.
Enlargement of a single frame from a cineangiocardiogram of a patient with tricuspid atresia. Note the right atrium, left atrium, left ventricle, and superior vena cava. The *arrow* is pointing to the expected location of the right ventricle, which is not opacified. *RA* = right atrium; *LA* = left atrium; *LV* = left ventricle; *SVC* = superior vena cava.

total anomalous pulmonary venous connection, and tetralogy of Fallot. The presence of dominant left ventricular hypertrophy in the ECG will virtually eliminate all of these lesions from serious consideration.

The major lesion presenting confusion is pulmonary atresia with an intact ventricular septum and a normal tricuspid valve. Blood does pass through the tricuspid valve into the right ventricle but then refluxes back to the right atrium, to follow the circulation of the patient

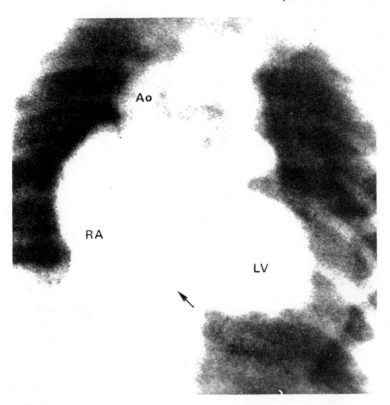

FIG 10–9.
Enlargement of a single frame from a cineangiocardiogram of a patient with tricuspid atresia, taken slightly later in systole than Figure 10–9. Note the appearance of the aorta. The right ventricular area *(arrow)* is narrowed but persists. *RA* = right atrium; *LV* = left ventricle; *Ao* = aorta.

with tricuspid atresia. Pulmonary atresia can be suspected if there are right-sided forces in the ECG as shown by the presence of normal or right-axis deviation and an R wave in V_1 and an S wave in $V_{5, 6}$. The echocardiogram can be of considerable assistance in this differential diagnosis. If the patient has pulmonary atresia, the tricuspid valve will be visualized, whereas if the diagnosis is tricuspid atresia, a nonfunctioning structure will be found at the expected location of the tricuspid valve.

PEARLS

1. There is no sex differentiation with this lesion.
2. Intense cyanosis in a newborn with left ventricular hypertrophy in the ECG strongly suggests the diagnosis.
3. Pulmonary atresia with intact ventricular septum should be ruled out, because the therapy of the two lesions may differ.
4. Without surgical intervention, early death can be anticipated.

11

Transposition of the Great Arteries

EMBRYOLOGY

Toward the end of the third week and into the fourth, the common trunk is divided into the pulmonary artery and the aorta. This is accomplished by a caudad spiral growth of the truncoconal ridges (Fig 11–1).

The mechanism behind this spiral growth is subject to several basic theories. The first suggests that the spiral motion of the blood from each potential ventricular chamber into the truncus arteriosus causes the septum to assume a corresponding spiral direction. This would result in the left ventricle emptying its blood into a vessel that would become the aorta and the right ventricle emptying its blood into a vessel that would become the pulmonary artery. A second theory suggests that as the bulbus cordis develops, it enlarges and rotates, carrying with it the truncoconal septum in such a way that the aorta will arise from the left ventricle and the pulmonary artery from the right ventricle. If there is disruption of either of these two mechanisms, the septum will grow in a straight caudad direction, disrupting the expected relationship between the great vessels and the ventricular chambers.

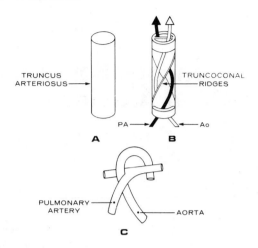

FIG 11–1.
Diagrammatic representation of the division of the truncus arteriosus **(A)** into the aorta and the pulmonary artery **(C)**. **B** shows the septation and the spiral direction of the pulmonary artery and the aorta. *PA* = pulmonary artery; *Ao* = aorta.

ANATOMY

By definition, when the great arteries are transposed, the aorta will arise from the anterior ventricle. This being a right ventricle, it will have an infundibulum, and the aortic valve and its sinuses will sit on top of that infundibulum. The normal continuity between the aortic and mitral valve rings will be lost. The pulmonary artery will arise from the posterior ventricle. This being a left ventricle, it will not have an infundibulum, and the pulmonary valves will have been drawn down inferiorly and posteriorly, putting the pulmonary valve ring in continuity with the mitral valve ring. The root of the aorta, therefore, will be anterior, superior, and rightward in its location, whereas the root of the pulmonary artery will be posterior, inferior, and leftward in its location (Fig 11–2).

Although the basic embryologic error that results in transposition of the great arteries may leave the remainder of the heart totally intact, lesions may coexist. The most commonly found additional defects are patent ductus arteriosus, ventricular septal defect, ventricular septal defect with subpulmonic stenosis, and, much less commonly, any

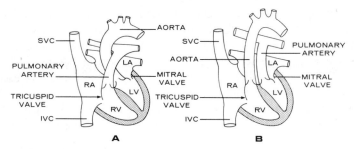

FIG 11–2.

Diagrammatic representation of the anatomical findings in a patient with transposition of the great arteries **(B)** compared with normal **(A).** (See text for explanation.) *IVC* = inferior vena cava; *SVC* = superior vena cava; *RA* = right atrium; *RV* = right ventricle; *LA* = left atrium; *LV* = left ventricle.

combination of the three. For the sake of simplicity, the remainder of this chapter is devoted to discussing transposition of the great arteries as it occurs with an intact ventricular septum, with a ventricular septal defect, or with a ventricular septal defect and subpulmonic stenosis.

TRANSPOSITION OF THE GREAT ARTERIES WITH INTACT VENTRICULAR SEPTUM

Hemodynamics

The patient with transposition of the great arteries with an intact ventricular septum has two parallel circuits and can be depicted conceptually in the mnemonic

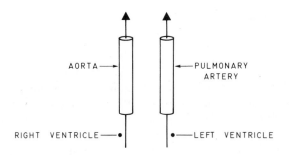

The arrows represent the blood flow from each ventricle into its respective great vessel. It should be noted that the right ventricle leads to the aorta and the left ventricle to the pulmonary artery. Although, for diagrammatic purposes, the great vessels are shown side by side, it must be remembered that in the patient they actually relate to each other in an anteroposterior direction. If the blood flow is followed with the mnemonic in mind, the effect on the various chambers and vessels of the heart can be demonstrated by the following diagram:

RIGHT ATRIUM ↑	LEFT ATRIUM →
RIGHT VENTRICLE ↑	LEFT VENTRICLE →
AORTA →	MAIN PULMONARY ARTERY →
	PULMONARY VESSELS ↑

The arrows represent alteration in the size of a chamber or a vessel as follows:

→ Unchanged
↑ Increased

This information can be translated to the chest roentgenogram, where one would expect cardiomegaly, with an enlarged right atrium and right ventricle. Because the great vessels relate in an anteroposterior direction, the mediastinum will be narrow. The blood flow to the lungs normally is increased, and therefore the vascular markings would be increased (Fig 11–3). With early diagnosis, however, it may be entirely normal. The electrocardiogram (ECG) would be expected to show right ventricular hypertrophy and perhaps right atrial hypertrophy, but, again, with early diagnosis it may be entirely normal (Fig 11–4).

Clinical Application

The patient essentially has two independent parallel circuits, and life is dependent on some intermixing of those two circuits. This occurs through the foramen ovale and the ductus arteriosus. Physiologic closure of both would result in sudden death. Depending on the degree of intermixing through the ductus arteriosus and the foramen ovale, the infant will be either minimally cyanotic or intensely blue. The bi-

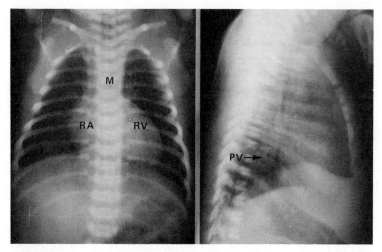

FIG 11–3.

Chest roentgenograms of an infant with transposition of the great arteries. Note the slightly enlarged right atrium and right ventricle. The mediastinum is narrow. The pulmonary vessels are somewhat increased. The overall cardiac size is slightly larger than normal. *RA* = right atrium; *RV* = right ventricle; *M* = mediastinum; *PV* = pulmonary vessels.

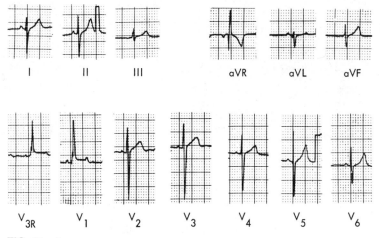

FIG 11–4.

Electrocardiogram of an infant with transposition of the great arteries. The salient features are the dominant S_1 and R/S_{aVF}—right axis deviation. Also present are a dominant R wave in V_1 and S wave in $V_{5,6}$, interpretable as right ventricular hypertrophy. The T wave in V_1 is also upright.

directional flow is dependent on subtle changes in systemic and pulmonary resistances and usually is in such low volume as not to cause a murmur. Even though there are two great vessels and two sets of valves, the common auscultatory finding is that of a single intensified second sound. This usually represents closure of the aortic valve, which is close to the chest wall.

The diagnosis can be suspected in a male infant who has minimal to moderate cyanosis, no significant murmurs, and a single second sound. The chest roentgenogram will show cardiomegaly, a narrow mediastinum, and increased vascular markings. The ECG will show right ventricular hypertrophy and, possibly, right atrial hypertrophy. The two-dimensional echocardiogram in the parasternal short-axis view can very nicely demonstrate the two great arteries in cross section visualized as two circles. When compared with the expected circle of the aorta and outflow tract of the right ventricle as a tube, the diagnosis can accurately be established (Fig 11–5). Cardiac catheterization will then serve to further elaborate the diagnosis, demonstrating pe-

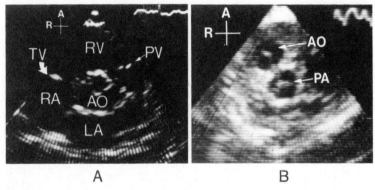

A   B

FIG 11–5.
Short-axis view of echocardiogram in a normal patient **(A)** and in a patient with *d*-transposition of the great arteries **(B).** Note in **B** the two circles related in an anteroposterior position compared with the single circle of the aorta and the pulmonary valve in the normal echocardiogram. *A* = anterior; *R* = right; *RV* = right ventricle; *TV* = tricuspid valve; *RA* = right atrium; *LA* = left atrium; *AO* = aorta; *PV* = pulmonary valve; *PA* = pulmonary artery. (From Silverman NH, Snider AR: *Two-Dimensional Echocardiography in Congenital Heart Disease.* Norwalk, Conn, Appleton-Century-Crofts, 1982, p 168. Used by permission.)

ripheral desaturation, systemic pressures in the right ventricle, the aorta arising from the right ventricle, and the pulmonary artery arising from the left ventricle (Table 11–1). Cineangiocardiography will show the great vessel relationship (Figs 11–6 and 11–7). In the newborn there has not yet been sufficient time for resolution of the pulmonary vascular bed, and the pressure in the left ventricle, which faces pulmonary resistance, will be essentially the same as the right ventricle, which faces systemic resistance.

Parenthetically, it should be reiterated that frequently in the first day of life, the roentgenogram and ECG will not have assumed the classic findings as discussed earlier. They may be very close to normal, making the diagnosis much more elusive. Within a few short days, however, if an index of suspicion is maintained, evidence for the existence of congenital heart disease will mount, and echocardiography and cardiac catheterization will permit the establishment of an accurate diagnosis.

TABLE 11–1.

Idealized Cardiac Catheterization Data in a Newborn With Transposition of the Great Arteries and Intact Ventricular Septum*

Site	Pressure (mm Hg)		Oxygen Saturation (%)	
	Normal	Patient	Normal	Patient
Superior vena cava			70	48
Inferior vena cava			74	52
Right atrium	a = 5 v = 4 m = 4	a = 5 v = 4 m = 4	72	50
Right ventricle	60/2	60/2	72	50
Aorta	60/40	60/40	97	50
Left atrium	a = 5 v = 7 m = 6	a = 5 v = 7 m = 6	97	97
Left ventricle	60/2	60/2	97	97
Main pulmonary artery	60/40	60/40	72	97

*The salient feature is decreased oxygen saturation in the right side of the heart as well as the aorta. The pressure in both the right and left ventricles is systemic in height. The order of the sites indicates that the aorta arises from the right ventricle and the main pulmonary artery from the left ventricle.

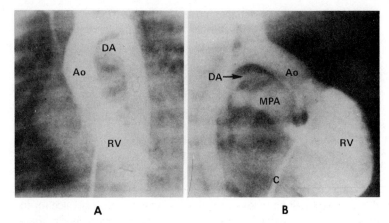

A   **B**

FIG 11–6.
Enlargements of two 35-mm cineangiocardiographic frames in a patient with transposition of the great arteries. Note that the aorta arises from the right ventricle and that the main pulmonary artery fills from the ductus arteriosus. **A,** anteroposterior projection; **B,** lateral projection. C = catheter; *RV* = right ventricle; *Ao* = aorta; *DA* = ductus arteriosus; *MPA* = main pulmonary artery.

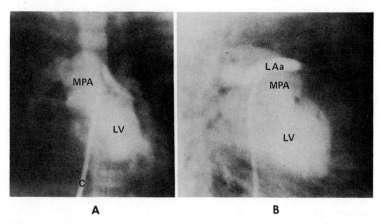

A   **B**

FIG 11–7.
Enlargements of two 35-mm cineangiocardiographic frames in a patient with transposition of the great arteries. Note that the main pulmonary artery arises from the left ventricle. **A,** anteroposterior projection; **B,** lateral projection. C = catheter; *LV* = left ventricle; *MPA* = main pulmonary artery; *LAa* = left atrial appendage.

TRANSPOSITION OF THE GREAT ARTERIES WITH VENTRICULAR SEPTAL DEFECT

Hemodynamics

This combination of defects can be demonstrated in the mnemonic

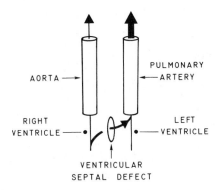

The arrows represent the blood flow from each ventricle into its respective great vessel plus right-to-left flow through the ventricular septal defect. If the blood flow is followed with the mnemonic in mind, the effect on the various chambers and vessels of the heart can be demonstrated by the following diagram:

RIGHT ATRIUM → ↑   LEFT ATRIUM → ↑
RIGHT VENTRICLE ↑   LEFT VENTRICLE → ↑
AORTA →   MAIN PULMONARY ARTERY → ↑
PULMONARY VESSELS ↑

The arrows represent changes in the size of a chamber or a vessel as follows:

→ Unchanged
↑ Increased

Translated to the chest roentgenogram, one would expect to find a normal or slightly enlarged right atrium, an enlarged right ventricle, and a normal to enlarged left atrium and left ventricle. Because the great vessels relate in an anteroposterior direction, the mediastinum would be narrow. The pulmonary vascular markings would be increased. These findings are so similar to those in a patient with an intact ventricular septum that Figure 11–3 remains representative. The ECG would be expected to show biventricular hypertrophy. The degree of left ventricular hypertrophy is dependent on the size of the ventricular septal defect and the degree of pulmonary vascular resistance. Despite these theoretic and practical statements, right ventricular hypertrophy generally is seen (see Fig 11–4).

Clinical Application

Because the pulmonary resistance at birth generally is equal to the systemic resistance, there is little flow across the ventricular septal defect. The patient with transposition of the great arteries with ventricular septal defect, therefore, may be indistinguishable from one without a ventricular septal defect. It is only after there is some drop in pulmonary resistance through natural maturation that the clinical picture will change. As this resistance drops, shunting can take place through the defect. In this instance, because the left ventricle relates to the pulmonary circuit, it will have the lower pressure and the shunting will be from the right ventricle to the left ventricle. Then a holosystolic murmur will occur at the fourth interspace to the left of the sternum, and if loud enough, it will be accompanied by a thrill. The flow through the ventricular septal defect will pass through the pulmonary vessels and be returned to the left atrium. This increased volume will enlarge the size of the atrium, stretch the foramen ovale, and permit the shunting of oxygenated blood into the right atrium. It should be apparent that this combination of anatomical and physiologic communications will permit the delivery of venous blood to the lungs and oxygenated blood to the body. It also must be stated that the increased flow of blood under an increased head of pressure to the pulmonary circuit places the lung at risk for the development of pulmonary vascular disease. The remainder of the examination will be similar to that in a patient with an intact ventricular septum and will not be repeated here. This diagnosis can be suspected in a male infant who has findings suggestive of transposition of the great arteries but who has holosystolic murmur at the fourth interspace to the left of the sternum. The chest roentgenogram would show cardiomegaly, a narrow mediastinum, and increased vascular markings, and the ECG would show dominant right ventricular hypertrophy. A two-dimensional echocardiogram in the parasternal short-axis view will confirm the diagnosis (see Fig 11–5). With the use of additional views, the ventricular septal defect can also be visualized (not demonstrated). Cardiac catheterization will demonstrate peripheral desaturation, systemic pressures in the right ventricle, the aorta arising from the right ventricle, and more specifically, evidence of left-to-right shunting at the atrial level and right-to-left shunting at the ventricular level. Cineangiocardiography would demonstrate the ventricular septal defect and the great vessel abnormality.

TRANSPOSITION OF THE GREAT ARTERIES WITH VENTRICULAR SEPTAL DEFECT AND SUBPULMONIC STENOSIS

Hemodynamics

The patient with this combination of defects has markedly diminished blood flow to the lungs and can be depicted in the mnemonic

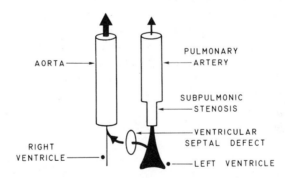

The arrows represent the blood flow from each ventricle into its respective great vessel. The smaller arrow leaving the pulmonary artery suggests the diminished blood flow to the lungs. The narrowed part of the pulmonary artery represents the subpulmonic stenosis. The heavy base of the arrow below the pulmonary artery suggests the increased pressure in the left ventricle. The shunting through the ventricular septal defect is shown as a heavy arrow passing through it and entering the aorta, with a resultant greater flow through the aorta, as shown by the heavier arrow leaving that great vessel. If the blood flow is followed with the mnemonic in mind, the effect on the various chambers and vessels of the heart can be demonstrated by the following diagram:

RIGHT ATRIUM ↑   LEFT ATRIUM →
RIGHT VENTRICLE ↑   LEFT VENTRICLE ↑
AORTA →   MAIN PULMONARY ARTERY → ↓
PULMONARY VESSELS ↓

The arrows represent the effect on the heart and great vessels as follows:

→ Unchanged
↑ Increased
↓ Decreased

These changes can be translated to the chest roentgenogram, where one would expect to find cardiomegaly with right atrial and biventricular enlargement. The mediastinum would be narrow because of the anteroposterior relationship of the great vessels. The pulmonary vascular markings would be diminished. Aside from the diminished pulmonary vascular markings, the findings are similar enough to those seen in a patient with an intact ventricular septum to permit Figure 11–3 to be representative. Although theoretically the ECG should show biventricular hypertrophy, the usual finding is only right ventricular hypertrophy (see Fig 11–4).

Clinical Application

With this combination, the subpulmonic stenosis creates a higher resistance to pulmonary flow than systemic flow, thus permitting the delivery of more oxygenated blood from the left ventricle through the ventricular septal defect to the aorta. One might then expect the patient to become less cyanotic. However, as the pulmonary stenosis becomes more severe, the patient actually becomes more cyanotic. With the increase in pulmonary stenosis, the resistance of flow to the lungs increases and there is a diminution in pulmonary flow. This results in a decrease in left atrial pressure, which, with the consistently elevated right atrial pressure, will cause a right-to-left shunt at the level of the atria. The mixing of poorly oxygenated systemic venous blood with the well-oxygenated pulmonary venous blood will result in an overall diminished saturation of blood delivered to the left ventricle. The cycle repeats itself to such a degree that blood leaving the left ventricle through the ventricular septal defect to the aorta becomes progressively lower in saturation.

The basic physical findings will be similar to those in any other patient with transposition of the great arteries. There will be, in addition, a systolic ejection murmur high along the left sternal border representing flow through the subpulmonic stenosis.

The diagnosis can be suspected in an infant who has findings suggestive of transposition of the great arteries but who is more cyanotic and has an ejection systolic murmur along the left sternal border, a chest roentgenogram with cardiomegaly, a narrow mediastinum and decreased vascular markings, and an ECG with dominant right ventricular hypertrophy. A two-dimensional echocardiogram in the parasternal short-axis view will demonstrate the abnormal relationship of the great arteries, thereby establishing the basic diagnosis. Demonstration of the subpulmonic stenosis and the ventricular septal defect is more difficult, but possible (not illustrated). Cardiac catheterization will demonstrate peripheral desaturation, systemic pressures in both ventricles, the origin of the aorta from the right ventricle, the origin of the pulmonary artery from the left ventricle, and, if entered, low pressures in the pulmonary artery. Cineangiocardiography would identify the ventricular septal defect, the subpulmonic stenosis, and the great vessel relationship.

DIFFERENTIAL DIAGNOSIS

The patient with transposition of the great arteries must be differentiated from one having truncus arteriosus, total anomalous pulmonary venous connection, tricuspid atresia, and, rarely, tetralogy of Fallot (note that all of these lesions begin with the letter "t"). Each of these lesions is discussed in detail in its respective chapter.

The patient with truncus arteriosus is similar in that cyanosis appears at about the same time and the second sound is single; however, it differs in that murmurs are rather consistently present and frequently continuous in character, the chest roentgenogram shows a wide mediastinum and cardiomegaly, and the ECG shows biventricular hypertrophy. Cardiac catheterization will demonstrate the single great artery, completing the differential diagnosis.

The patient with total anomalous pulmonary venous connection with obstruction will be easily differentiated on the basis of a small heart on roentgenogram. One without obstruction will have a well-split second sound, an ejection systolic murmur along the left sternal border, and cardiomegaly on roentgenogram.

The patient with tricuspid atresia will also be cyanotic, but the presence of left axis deviation and left ventricular hypertrophy on the ECG will quickly make the differential diagnosis clear.

The patient with tetralogy of Fallot, although included in the differential diagnosis on the basis of cyanosis, is easily differentiated. The cyanosis occurs later in life, murmurs are heard consistently, and the chest roentgenogram shows diminished vascular markings and a boot-shaped heart and lacks a narrow mediastinum.

PEARLS

1. Transposition of the great arteries is more common in males than in females.
2. The cyanosis may be quite subtle.
3. The diagnosis on the first day of life may be extremely difficult, and a high index of suspicion must persist.
4. The birth weight of patients with transposition of the great arteries usually is normal or greater than normal.
5. Early diagnosis is essential, because when the ductus arteriosus closes, sudden death occurs.
6. The terms *d*-transposition of the great arteries, simple transposition, and transposition of the great arteries are interchangeable.

12 | Truncus Arteriosus

EMBRYOLOGY

Toward the end of the third week and into the fourth, the common trunk normally is divided into the pulmonary artery and the aorta. This is accomplished by the development of the truncoconal ridges, which grow caudad in a spiral fashion, resulting in the posterolateral takeoff of the aorta and the anteromedial takeoff of the pulmonary artery (Fig 12–1). This septum fuses with the bulbar ridges, which, in turn, participate with the endocardial cushions and membranous proliferation from the ventricular septum to form the definitive closure of the interventricular septum (Fig 12–2).

ANATOMY

If the septation of the common trunk fails to take place, a single great vessel persists, which receives blood from both the left and right ventricles. Since the truncal septum participates in the final closure of

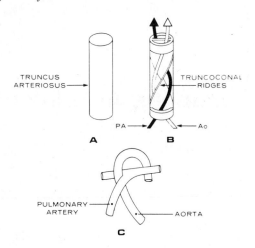

FIG 12–1.
Diagrammatic representation of the division of the truncus arteriosus **(A)** into the aorta and the pulmonary artery **(C)**. **B,** septation and spiral direction of the pulmonary artery and the aorta. *PA* = pulmonary artery; *Ao* = aorta.

the ventricular septum, there must be a ventricular septal defect in conjunction with the common trunk (one of the rare "musts" in medicine). As in most of pediatric cardiology, variations on the theme have occurred, and truncus arteriosus has been subdivided into four basic anatomical varieties. Type I (Fig 12–3, A) has a common trunk

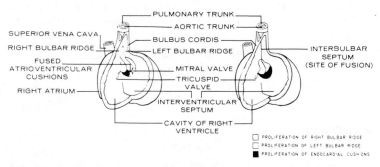

FIG 12–2.
Diagrammatic representation of the final fusion of the ventricular septum and its relationship to the bulbar ridges.

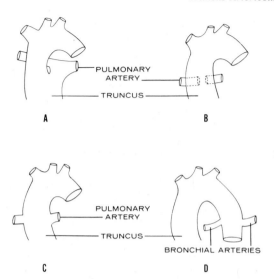

FIG 12–3.
Classification of truncus arteriosus. **A,** type I; **B,** type II; **C,** type III; **D,** type IV.
(See text for explanation.)

arising from the heart and a partial septation of that trunk giving
rise to the dominant aorta and the right and left pulmonary arteries
as shown. Type II (Fig 12–3, B) has pulmonary arteries that arise
from the posterior surface of the common trunk. Type III (Fig 12–3,
C) has pulmonary arteries arising from the lateral walls of the
common trunk. Type IV (Fig 12–3, D) has no pulmonary arteries
at all but, rather, bronchial arteries arising from the descending
aorta.

HEMODYNAMICS

Regardless of the anatomical variety, the patient with a truncus arteriosus has a common outlet for both right and left ventricular output.
The blood flow to the lungs, however, will vary from increased to diminished, depending on the specific variety. The overall concept is
shown in the mnemonic

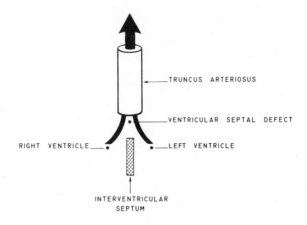

The arrows represent blood flow from each ventricle into the common trunk.

In the first three types of truncus arteriosus, pulmonary arteries are present and arise in one way or another from the common trunk. If this is kept in mind and the flow followed, the effect on the heart can be demonstrated by the following diagram:

RIGHT ATRIUM →   LEFT ATRIUM →
RIGHT VENTRICLE ↑   LEFT VENTRICLE ↑
BRANCH PULMONARY ARTERIES ↑   TRUNK ↑
PULMONARY VESSELS ↑

The arrows represent alteration in the size of a chamber or a vessel as follows:

→ Unchanged
↑ Increased

This information can be translated to the chest roentgenogram, where one would expect cardiomegaly, biventricular enlargement, and a wide mediastinum. The pulmonary arteries frequently arise in a more superior location from the trunk, and this may be seen on the roentgenogram. The vascular markings would be increased (Fig 12–4). The electrocardiogram (ECG) would show biventricular hypertrophy (Fig 12–5).

In the fourth type of truncus arteriosus, no pulmonary artery is

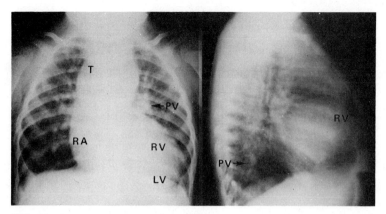

FIG 12-4.

Chest roentgenograms of a 1-year-old patient with type II truncus arteriosus. Note the cardiomegaly, wide mediastinum caused by the large trunk, the enlarged right atrium, right ventricle, and left ventricle. The pulmonary vessels are increased. T = trunk; RA = right atrium; RV = right ventricle; LV = left ventricle; PV = pulmonary vessels.

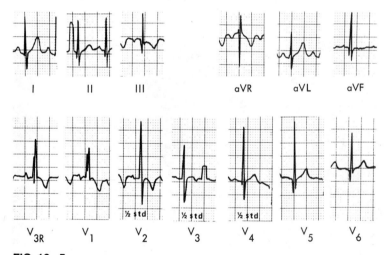

FIG 12-5.

Electrocardiogram of a 1-year-old patient with type II truncus arteriosus showing combined ventricular hypertrophy. The salient features are a dominant R wave in leads V_1 and $V_{5,6}$ and tall complexes in leads $V_{2,3,4}$.

present and pulmonary circulation is through dilated bronchial arteries. If this is kept in mind, the flow as represented in the mnemonic would affect the heart as demonstrated in the following diagram:

RIGHT ATRIUM → ↑   LEFT ATRIUM →
RIGHT VENTRICLE ↑   LEFT VENTRICLE →
PULMONARY ARTERIES ○   AORTA →
PULMONARY VESSELS ↓

The arrows represent alteration in the size of a chamber or a vessel as follows:

→ Unchanged
↑ Increased
↓ Decreased
○ Absent

Once more translating this to the chest roentgenogram, one would expect to find right ventricular enlargement, an absence of the pulmonary artery bulge on the left border of the heart, and very diminished pulmonary vessels (Fig 12–6). The ECG would show dominant right ventricular hypertrophy (Fig 12–7).

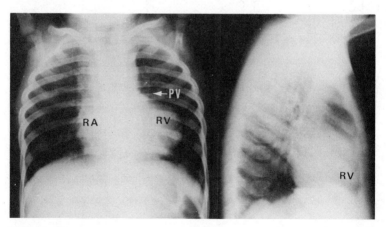

FIG 12–6.
Chest roentgenograms of a 1-year-old patient with type IV truncus arteriosus. The salient features are enlargement of the right atrium and right ventricle and diminished pulmonary vessels. *RA* = right atrium; *RV* = right ventricle; *PV* = pulmonary vessels.

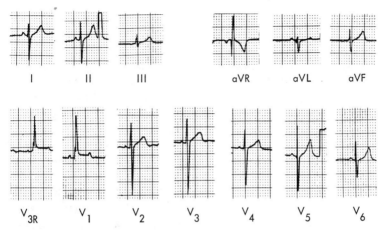

FIG 12–7.
Electrocardiogram of a 1-year-old patient with type IV truncus arteriosus. The salient features are the dominant S_1 and R/S_{aVF} right axis deviation. Also present are a dominant R wave in V_1 and S wave in $V_{5, 6}$, interpretable as right ventricular hypertrophy. The T wave in V_1 is also upright.

CLINICAL APPLICATION

Although each anatomical variation of truncus arteriosus will have subtle differences, there is sufficient similarity to permit presenting the entire panorama under a single subtitle noting the differences rather than going to the extent of totally separate presentations.

Because of the large dilated trunk, the onset of systole may be introduced with an ejection click. This will be followed by a systolic murmur, more ejection in quality than anything else, and varying in intensity from grade II/VI to, rarely, grade IV/VI. It is heard at about the fourth interspace to the left of the sternum. It may well transmit along the great vessels of the aorta and much less frequently into the pulmonary arteries. At times, a continuous murmur can be heard on the anterior chest. The diastolic component may be related to flow into the pulmonary arteries during the diastolic phase of the cardiac cycle. Because there is a single set of leaflets—three or four—and not two separate sets of semilunar valves, the second sound can be anticipated to be single. This is a very consistent finding. The blood flow into the lungs will be variable, depending on the pulmonary resistance. If this flow happens to be significant, the return to the left atrium may result in a mid-diastolic filling sound as it passes across the mitral valve. Also, continuous murmurs may be heard across the back as well as the anterior aspect of the chest because of bronchial flow.

The patient with truncus arteriosus is consistently cyanotic. However, the degree of cyanosis may vary from minimal (when there is adequate pulmonary flow) to intense (when the flow is through small bronchial arteries). If there is significant pulmonary flow (types I, II, and III), the burden on the left side of the heart can result in early congestive heart failure. The usual symptoms of cough and signs of tachypnea with dyspnea, tachycardia, and hepatomegaly will be seen.

With a combination of views, the two-dimensional echocardiogram is capable of demonstrating the truncus arteriosus. The parasternal long-axis view will show the large trunk overriding the ventricular septum with its defect in the membranous portion (Fig 12–8). Following the trunk cephalad, the origin of the branches of the pulmonary artery can be imaged (not illustrated). This information can be supplemented by cardiac catheterization, which will demonstrate a decrease

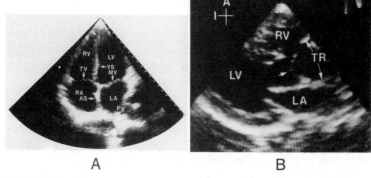

A   B

FIG 12–8.
Parasternal long-axis echocardiogram in a normal patient **(A)** and in a patient with truncus arteriosus **(B).** Note in **B** the overriding of the ventricular septum by the truncal vessel and the *little arrow* demonstrating the reversed doming of the truncal valves. A = anterior; I = inferior; RV = right ventricle; S = septum; LV = left ventricle; LA = left atrium; AO = aorta; TR = truncus. (From Silverman NH, Snider AR: *Two-Dimensional Echocardiography in Congenital Heart Disease.* Norwalk, Conn, Appleton-Century-Crofts, 1982, p 158. Used by permission.)

in oxygen saturation in the trunk and the pulmonary arteries. Pressures in the right ventricle and the pulmonary artery will be systemic in height. Minimal elevation of right and left atrial pressures can be expected (Table 12–1). Cineangiocardiography would demonstrate the large common trunk and the origin of the pulmonary arteries (Fig 12–9).

If there is insufficient pulmonary flow (type IV), the patient tends not to go into heart failure but, rather, to be exposed to the risks of severe hypoxia. These are acidosis and, more threateningly, hypoxic spells. During cardiac catheterization, the pulmonary artery cannot be entered and systemic pressures in the right ventricle and systemic desaturation will be found (Table 12–2). Angiocardiography will confirm the absence of a main pulmonary artery and the presence of some form of bronchial circulation (Fig 12–10).

The diagnosis of the first three types of truncus arteriosus can be suspected in an infant who is cyanotic and has a single second sound,

TABLE 12–1.

Idealized Cardiac Catheterization Data in a Young Child With Type II Truncus Arteriosus*

Site	Pressure (mm Hg)		Oxygen Saturation (%)	
	Normal	Patient	Normal	Patient
Superior vena cava			70	60
Inferior vena cava			74	68
Right atrium	a = 5 v = 3 m = 4	a = 9 v = 6 m = 5	72	64
Right ventricle	25/2	100/8	72	64
Pulmonary artery	25/12	100/40	72	76
Left atrium	a = 5 v = 7 m = 6	a = 7 v = 12 m = 10	97	97
Left ventricle	100/5	100/4	97	97
Aorta (trunk)	100/55	100/55	97	76

*The salient features are slightly elevated pressures in the right atrium, systemic pressures in the right ventricle and the pulmonary artery, and desaturation in the trunk and the pulmonary artery.

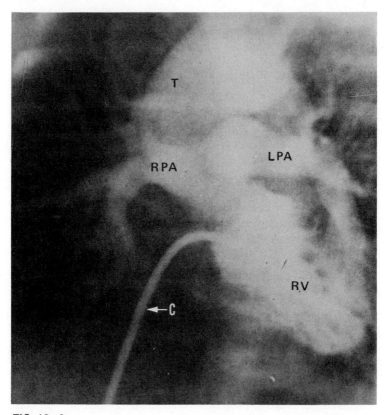

FIG 12–9.
An enlargement of a single 35-mm frame taken from a cineangiocardiogram performed on a 1-year-old patient with type II truncus arteriosus. The tip of the catheter is in the right ventricle. The salient features are the enlarged trunk and the presence of a right pulmonary artery and a left pulmonary artery, which arise from the posterior aspect of the trunk. *C* = catheter; *RV* = right ventricle; *T* = trunk; *RPA* = right pulmonary artery; *LPA* = left pulmonary artery.

murmurs varying from minimal to continuous, a chest roentgenogram showing cardiomegaly, displaced pulmonary arteries, and increased vascular markings, and an ECG showing combined ventricular hypertrophy.

The patient with the fourth type will be more deeply cyanotic, have much less of a murmur on the anterior chest but significant wide-

TABLE 12–2.

Idealized Cardiac Catheterization Data in a Young Child With Type IV
Truncus Arteriosus*

Site	Pressure (mm Hg) Normal	Pressure (mm Hg) Patient	Oxygen Saturation (%) Normal	Oxygen Saturation (%) Patient
Superior vena cava			70	43
Inferior vena cava			74	49
Right atrium	a = 5 v = 3 m = 4	a = 12 v = 7 m = 9	72	45
Right ventricle	25/2	100/5	72	45
Main pulmonary artery	25/12	Not entered	72	Not entered
Left atrium	a = 5 v = 7 m = 6	a = 5 v = 7 m = 6	97	97
Left ventricle	100/5	100/5	97	97
Aorta (trunk)	100/55	100/55	97	65

*The salient features are an increase in pressure in the right atrium, systemic pressures in the right ventricle, the inability to enter a pulmonary artery, desaturation in the right atrium and ventricle, and desaturation in the aorta.

spread continuous murmurs over the posterior chest, a single second sound, a roentgenogram with diminished vascular markings, and an ECG showing right ventricular hypertrophy.

DIFFERENTIAL DIAGNOSIS

The patient with truncus arteriosus must be differentiated from one having transposition of the great arteries, total anomalous pulmonary venous connection, tricuspid atresia, and tetralogy of Fallot (note that all of these lesions begin with the letter "t"). Each of them is discussed in detail in its respective chapter.

The patient with transposition of the great arteries is similar in that the cyanosis appears early in infancy and the second sound is single but differs in that murmurs generally are absent and the chest roentgenogram shows a narrow mediastinum with cardiomegaly and

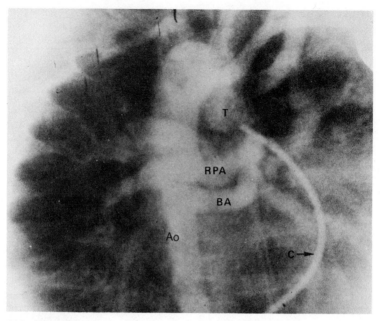

FIG 12–10.
An enlargement of a single 35-mm frame taken from a cineangiocardiogram performed on a 1-year-old patient with type IV truncus arteriosus. The tip of the catheter is in the ascending trunk. The salient features are the presence of a bronchial artery arising from the descending aorta and the filling of the right pulmonary artery from the bronchial artery. *C* = catheter; *T* = trunk; *BA* = bronchial artery; *Ao* = aorta; *RPA* = right pulmonary artery.

the ECG shows right ventricular hypertrophy. Echocardiography and, if necessary, cardiac catheterization will permit the differentiation.

The patient with total anomalous pulmonary venous connection with obstruction will be easily differentiated on the basis of a small heart on roentgenogram. One without obstruction will have a well-split second sound, an ejection systolic murmur along the left sternal border, and cardiomegaly on roentgenogram.

The patient with tricuspid atresia will only momentarily be considered on the basis of cyanosis. The presence of dominant left ventricular hypertrophy on the ECG will quickly make the differential diagnosis clear.

The patient with classic tetralogy of Fallot will have a more typical ejection systolic murmur at the second and third left interspace and on echocardiography a demonstrable right ventricular outflow tract and main pulmonary artery originating from it. However, the extreme variation of tetralogy—pulmonary atresia with ventricular septal defect—will be more difficult. The echocardiogram can demonstrate the confluence of miniscule pulmonary arteries, which would be absent in the type IV truncus.

PEARLS

1. Splitting of the second sound rules out truncus arteriosus.
2. There is no sex difference.
3. A right aortic arch is seen frequently.

13 | Total Anomalous Pulmonary Venous Connection

EMBRYOLOGY

At about the third week of gestation, the pulmonary venous drainage develops. The lung buds are in communication with the splanchnic plexus, which, in turn, is connected to the umbilical vitelline veins and the cardinal veins (Fig 13–1, A). At the same time, in the common atrium, there is an outpouching of a structure known as the common pulmonary vein, which grows to join the splanchnic plexus (Fig 13–1, B). The cardinal veins and the umbilical vitelline veins then lose their connections with the splanchnic plexus. This leaves the pulmonary veins draining into the left atrium through the common pulmonary vein (Fig 13–1, C). There is gradual absorption of the common pulmonary vein into the body of the left atrium, leading to the expected final relationship of four pulmonary veins draining into the left atrium proper (Fig 13–1, D).

ANATOMY

Any disruption of this mechanism will result in an obligatory circuitous pathway from the common pulmonary vein to the heart. Four

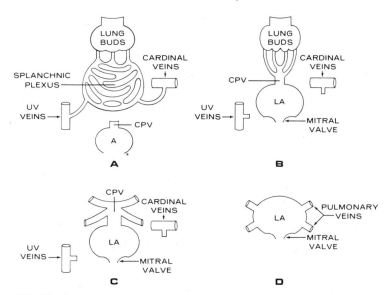

FIG 13–1.
Diagrammatic representation of the embryologic development of the pulmonary venous drainage. **A–D,** various stages of development are shown. (See text for explanation.) *UV VEINS* = umbilical vitelline veins; *A* = common atrium; *CPV* = common pulmonary vein; *LA* = left atrium.

anomalous pathways are commonly seen. The first is from the common pulmonary vein through a vertical vein into the innominate vein to the right superior vena cava and into the right atrium (Fig 13–2, A). The second is from the common pulmonary vein into the coronary sinus and then to the right atrium (Fig 13–2, B). The third is direct drainage into the right atrium as the result of absorption of the common pulmonary vein as four distinct pulmonary veins into that atrium (Fig 13–2, C). The fourth is from the common pulmonary vein inferiorly into the portal vein, which reaches the right atrium via the ductus venosus and the inferior vena cava (Fig 13–2, D).

Each of these communications can occur without any obstruction along the pulmonary venous pathway and be classified as total anomalous pulmonary venous connection without obstruction. Each of the communications can occur with obstruction along the pulmonary venous pathway and be classified as total anomalous pulmonary

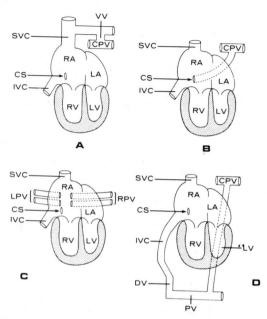

FIG 13–2.
Diagrammatic representation of the anatomical variations of total anomalous pulmonary venous connection. (See text for explanation.) *SVC* = superior vena cava; *IVC* = inferior vena cava; *RA* = right atrium; *CS* = coronary sinus; *RV* = right ventricle; *LA* = left atrium; *LV* = left ventricle; *CPV* = common pulmonary vein; *VV* = vertical vein; *LPV* = left pulmonary veins; *RPV* = right pulmonary veins; *PV* = portal vein; *DV* = ductus venosus.

venous connection with obstruction. The presence or absence of obstruction so affects the entire clinical picture that separation into the two major classifications for further discussion is prudent at this point.

TOTAL ANOMALOUS PULMONARY VENOUS CONNECTION WITH OBSTRUCTION

Hemodynamics

The obstruction in the pulmonary venous channel raises the pulmonary venous pressure, causes the pulmonary vascular resistance to rise, and results in pulmonary artery hypertension, placing a further pressure burden on the right ventricle. Pulmonary edema may result from the severe increase in pulmonary vascular pressure. This concept is demonstrated in the mnemonic

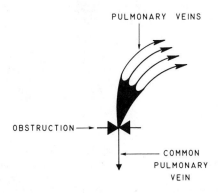

The single downward-pointing arrow being compressed by two horizontal arrows represents the obstruction of blood flow through the pulmonary vein. The multiple larger arrows pointing superiorly represent the backward pressure into the pulmonary veins. If the mnemonic is kept in mind, the effect on the heart can be demonstrated by the following diagram:

RIGHT ATRIUM →   LEFT ATRIUM ↓
RIGHT VENTRICLE → ↑   LEFT VENTRICLE ↓
MAIN PULMONARY ARTERY →   AORTA → ↓
PULMONARY VENOUS VESSELS ↑

The arrows represent alteration in the size of a chamber or a vessel as follows:

→ Unchanged
↑ Increased

This information can be translated to the chest roentgenogram, where one would expect to find a normal right atrium, a slightly enlarged right ventricle, a normal main pulmonary artery, and increased pulmonary venous markings. The left atrium and left ventricle would be small. The overall size of the heart is notably normal (Fig 13–3).

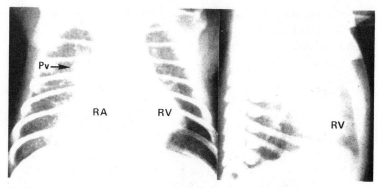

FIG 13–3.
Chest roentgenograms of an infant with total anomalous pulmonary venous drainage with obstruction. Note the overall small size of the heart and the punctate markings in the lungs representing pulmonary venous engorgement. *RA* = right atrium; *RV* = right ventricle; *Pv* = pulmonary venous engorgement.

The electrocardiogram (ECG) would show right ventricular hypertrophy (Fig 13–4).

Clinical Application

The clinical picture in such a patient is dependent on two sets of circumstances. The first is the amount of blood passing through the obstruction and where it goes, and the second, in an almost parenthetical sense, is the amount of blood that is unable to pass through the obstruction and where it goes.

Progressing forward first, the totally oxygenated blood that passes through the obstruction mixes with the venous blood returning from the superior and inferior venae cavae. The right atrial sample, therefore, will represent total venous mixing. The atrial septum is consistently patent, generally because of an anatomical atrial septal defect. As such, both the left atrium and the right ventricle will receive blood of equal saturation. Blood with the same degree of desaturation then will pass into the left ventricle and out the aorta, resulting in visible cyanosis. Since the volume of blood presented to the right atrium is relatively small, little turbulence will be created by passage of that blood across the tricuspid valve in diastole or out the pulmonary valve

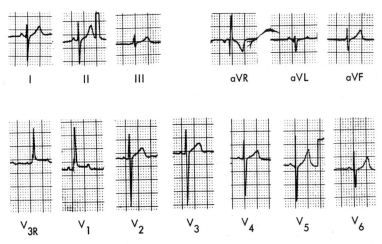

FIG 13–4.
Electrocardiogram of an infant with total anomalous pulmonary venous drainage with obstruction. The salient feature is the dominant S_I and R/S_{aVF} right-axis deviation. Also present are a dominant R wave in V_1 and S wave in $V_{5, 6}$, interpretable as right ventricular hypertrophy. The T wave in V_1 is also upright.

in systole. Therefore, murmurs may be nonexistent. In addition, right ventricular ejection time would not be prolonged, and the second sound would not be widely split.

That blood unable to pass through the obstruction will be collected in the pulmonary venous system and will cause pulmonary edema. Marked tachypnea and dyspnea will result. With time, secondary right ventricular hypertrophy and right ventricular failure will become apparent.

Depending on the degree of obstruction, these events will become known in the first day to the first week of life. The diagnosis can be suspected in an infant of average size—usually a male—who has minimal cyanosis, minimal or no murmurs, marked tachypnea and dyspnea, and, congestive heart failure. The ECG would show right ventricular hypertrophy, and the chest roentgenogram would show a relatively normal-sized heart but with increased pulmonary venous markings.

The diagnosis of total anomalous pulmonary venous connection with obstruction can be made by echocardiography but with difficulty.

If in the apical four-chamber view the pulmonary veins cannot be distinctly demonstrated as draining into the left atrium, an initial index of suspicion will be raised. In addition, in that view the right atrium and the right ventricle will be enlarged beyond normal. It then becomes the task to identify where the common pulmonary vein is. Frequently in the parasternal long-axis view the common vein can be demonstrated as an abnormal channel behind the left atrium (Fig 13–5). Knowing this will increase the efficiency with which the diagnosis and the details can be confirmed at cardiac catheterization. During the study one would expect to find comparable diminished oxygen saturations in each chamber and great artery, consistently elevated right ventricular pressures, and commonly elevated right atrial pressures. A localized increase in oxygen saturation will mark the entrance of the anomalous vein (Table 13–1). Ideally, cineangiocardiography will demonstrate the course of the anomalous vessel.

As was stated earlier, obstruction to the common pulmonary vein can occur whether its insertion is below the diaphragm into the inferior vena cava or portal system or above the diaphragm into the innominate vein. In the former instance, the obstruction can be caused by mechan-

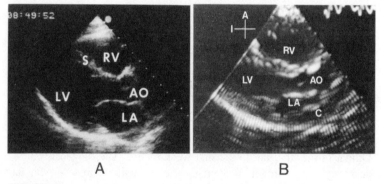

FIG 13–5.
Parasternal long-axis view of an echocardiogram in a normal patient **(A)** and in a patient with total anomalous pulmonary venous connection **(B).** Note in **B** the extra echo-free space representing the common pulmonary vein **(C)** lying posterior to the left atrium. *A* = anterior; *I* = inferior; *RV* = right ventricle; *S* = septum; *LV* = left ventricle; *LA* = left atrium; *AO* = aorta. (From Silverman NH, Snider AR: *Two-Dimensional Echocardiography in Congenital Heart Disease.* Norwalk, Conn, Appleton-Century-Crofts, 1982, p 206. Used by permission.)

TABLE 13-1.

Idealized Cardiac Catheterization Data in a Newborn With Total Anomalous Venous Connection Below the Diaphragm*

Site	Pressure (mm Hg)		Oxygen Saturation (%)	
	Normal	Patient	Normal	Patient
Common pulmonary vein			97	97
Superior vena cava			70	45
Inferior vena cava			74	70
Right atrium	a = 5 v = 3 m = 4	a = 10 v = 7 m = 8	72	55
Right ventricle	60/2	60/2	72	55
Main pulmonary artery	60/40	60/40	72	55
Left atrium	a = 5 v = 7 m = 6	a = 4 v = 6 m = 5	97	55
Left ventricle	60/2	60/2	97	55
Systemic artery	60/40	60/40	97	55

*The salient feature is an increase in oxygen saturation at the level of the inferior vena cava with final mixing in the right atrium. All other intracardiac values are identical. The pressures in the right atrium are elevated, and those in the right ventricle and main pulmonary artery are systemic in height. The elevated pressures in the right side of the heart, in the normal, are a reflection of the expected fetal pulmonary hypertension seen in the newborn.

ical constriction of the vein as it passes through the diaphragm or by physiologic obstruction of flow as it passes through the ductus venosus and the liver. When the insertion is above the diaphragm, the obstruction generally is mechanical and is the result of passage of the vessel between any two fixed structures. When obstruction is present, regardless of the course of the vein, the physiologic events are the same.

Differential Diagnosis

The patient with total anomalous pulmonary venous connection with obstruction must be differentiated from a patient having any other lesion causing cyanosis in infancy. This includes transposition of the great arteries, tricuspid atresia, truncus arteriosus, and tetralogy of Fallot.

The patient with transposition of the great arteries may present a confusing clinical picture at the outset of the examination. However, the increase in pulmonary vascular markings will be arterial in nature, the heart will be enlarged, and the mediastinum will be narrow. Since in the first days of life these findings will not be so obvious, a combination of echocardiography and cardiac catheterization generally will be necessary to make the differential diagnosis.

Tricuspid atresia will be eliminated in the differential diagnosis when it is apparent that the ECG indicates left axis deviation and left ventricular hypertrophy.

Classic tetralogy of Fallot rarely appears in the newborn period, but if so, the presence of markedly diminished pulmonary vascular markings assists in the differential diagnosis.

The patient with truncus arteriosus also will present a confusing clinical picture at the outset of the examination, but the chest roentgenogram will tend to show a somewhat enlarged heart with increased vascular markings. The presence of a systolic or a continuous murmur will be an additional aid. Cardiac catheterization and echocardiography will permit an accurate differentiation.

TOTAL ANOMALOUS PULMONARY VENOUS CONNECTION WITHOUT OBSTRUCTION

When obstruction of the common pulmonary vein is not present, it is most likely that the insertion of that vein is above the diaphragm. Theoretically, it is possible for the common vein to empty below the diaphragm without obstruction, and if so, the physical findings would be no different. However, because this is most uncommon, the remainder of this section deals with the events that follow the anomalous connection of the pulmonary venous drainage above the diaphragm into the innominate vein. The basic challenge to the heart is that of increased flow to the right atrium and is depicted in the mnemonic

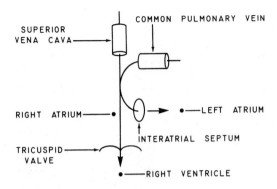

If the blood flow is followed with the mnemonic in mind, the effect on the various chambers and vessels can be demonstrated by the following diagram:

MEDIASTINUM ↑   PULMONARY VESSELS ↑
RIGHT ATRIUM ↑   LEFT ATRIUM → ↓
RIGHT VENTRICLE ↑   LEFT VENTRICLE → ↓
MAIN PULMONARY ARTERY ↑   AORTA →

The arrows represent alteration in the size of a chamber or a vessel as follows:

→ Unchanged
↑ Increased
↓ Decreased

This information can be translated to the chest roentgenogram, where one would expect an enlarged right atrium, right ventricle, and main pulmonary artery and increased pulmonary vascular markings. The left atrium would be small and the left ventricle small to normal. With time, the common pulmonary vein, which generally courses superiorly along the left side of the mediastinum, and the superior vena cava, which courses inferiorly along the right side of the mediastinum, will cause it to be wide and to give the appearance of a figure "8," or a snowman shape. This observation generally is not made until childhood (Fig 13–6). The ECG would show right ventricular hypertrophy and, at times, right atrial hypertrophy (see Fig 13–4).

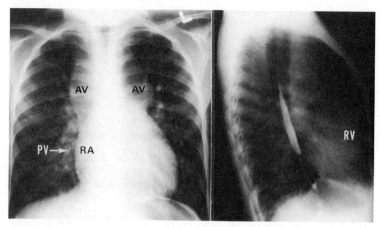

FIG 13–6.
Chest roentgenograms of a child with total anomalous pulmonary venous drainage above the diaphragm without obstruction. Note the increase in cardiac size with the prominent right atrium and increase in pulmonary vascular markings. The mediastinum is also wide because of the anomalous drainage and resembles a figure "8," or a snowman. *RA* = right atrium; *RV* = right ventricle; *AV* = anomalous vessels; *PV* = pulmonary vessels.

Clinical Application

The patient with total anomalous pulmonary venous connection without obstruction generally is asymptomatic in infancy. In fact, the entire clinical picture is quite reminiscent of that caused by an atrial septal defect. The entire pulmonary venous blood flow passes from the common pulmonary vein into the vertical vein and courses across to the superior vena cava. At each of these junctures, the systolic and diastolic flow can be heard as a high-pitched continuous murmur reminiscent of a venous hum (this is an uncommon finding). The pulmonary venous flow then augments the systemic venous return, delivering an extraordinary volume to the right atrium. Because of the obligatory interatrial communication, blood will flow both into the left atrium and across the tricuspid valve. The blood that passes across the valve may be heard as a mid-diastolic murmur. Right ventricular volume is increased, and right ventricular systolic ejection time is prolonged. The passage of blood across the pulmonary valve will be heard as an ejection systolic murmur varying in intensity from grade II to III, medium in pitch, and transmitting along the course of the pulmonary arterial vessels. The prolonged right ventricular ejection time will delay the closure of the pulmonary valve, resulting in a widely split second sound. The right ventricular volume overload is rather independent of venous return, and, therefore, fixed splitting of the second sound can be anticipated. The volume overload on the right side of the heart, which causes the right ventricular enlargement, will be palpable as a lift along the left sternal border.

The blood that passes into the left atrium remains desaturated (remember that the entire pulmonary venous return has already mixed with the systemic venous return), and the mixture eventually enters the aorta, accounting for the cyanosis generally seen.

The patient with total anomalous pulmonary venous connection is at risk for the development of pulmonary vascular disease. Its presence will be suggested by a progressive narrowing of the splitting of the second sound, an increase in intensity of the pulmonary component, and diminishing murmurs.

The diagnosis can be suspected in a patient—either male or female—who has relatively poor growth and development, a prominent left side of the chest, a right ventricular heave, a systolic ejection murmur high along the left chest, a mild diastolic murmur low along the left side of the chest, and a widely split second sound. A chest roentgenogram showing enlargement of the right atrium and ventricle and increased pulmonary vascular markings should raise the possibility of a left-to-right shunt. The presence of the snowman configuration should significantly point to the proper diagnosis. In the presence of visible cyanosis, the picture becomes complete. The ECG should lend support if it shows right ventricular hypertrophy. The diagnosis can generally be established by echocardiography using the same principles discussed in the early part of this chapter where total anomalous pulmonary venous connection with obstruction was presented. If indicated, the diagnosis can be finally confirmed with cardiac catheterization, during which one would find an increase in oxygen saturation in the superior vena cava, with essentially identical oxygen saturations being present in all four intracardiac chambers as well as in both great arteries (Table 13–2). Cineangiocardiography would demonstrate the

TABLE 13-2.

Idealized Cardiac Catheterization Data in a Young Child With Total Anomalous Pulmonary Venous Drainage Above the Diaphragm*

Site	Pressure (mm Hg)		Oxygen Saturation (%)	
	Normal	Patient	Normal	Patient
Common pulmonary vein			97	97
Superior vena cava			70	88
Inferior vena cava			74	60
Right atrium	a = 5 v = 3 m = 4	a = 10 v = 7 m = 8	72	80
Right ventricle	25/2	40/2	72	80
Main pulmonary artery	25/12	40/12	72	80
Left atrium	a = 5 v = 7 m = 6	a = 4 v = 6 m = 5	97	80
Left ventricle	100/2	100/2	97	80
Systemic artery	100/60	100/60	97	80

*The salient feature is an oxygen saturation in the superior vena cava that is greater than that in the inferior vena cava. There is final mixing, with relative desaturation in the right atrium and identical values in all other chambers and both great arteries. The pressures in the right atrium are elevated, as are those in the right ventricle and the main pulmonary artery.

absence of any pulmonary venous connection directly to the left atrium and might well show the anomalous vessel.

Differential Diagnosis

The patient with total anomalous pulmonary venous connection without obstruction must be differentiated from one having a large atrial septal defect, a ventricular septal defect, truncus arteriosus, and an atrioventricular canal.

The patient with an atrial septal defect will have similar clinical findings but will not be cyanotic either visibly or chemically. The presence of a wide mediastinum on roentgenogram will aid in the differential diagnosis.

If the patient with a ventricular septal defect has a classic grade

IV/VI holosystolic murmur, the differential diagnosis will be easy. If the patient has the Eisenmenger complex, peripheral desaturation will lend a note of confusion, but the absence of a snowman appearance on the heart will be helpful. Echocardiography and, if necessary, cardiac catheterization will permit an accurate differential diagnosis.

A truncus arteriosus will present the most confusing clinical findings in that the mediastinum may be wide and peripheral desaturation is consistently present. However, a single second sound will virtually establish the correct diagnosis. If necessary, echocardiography or cardiac catheterization (or both) and cineangiocardiography can finalize the differential diagnosis.

Diagnosis of an atrioventricular canal will be confusing in that the clinical picture may be similar but the cardiac silhouette on roentgenogram will be significantly greater and the ECG will show abnormal left axis deviation and biventricular hypertrophy. If necessary, cardiac catheterization can finalize the differential diagnosis.

PEARLS

1. Patients with obstruction tend to be males, whereas those without obstruction may be of either sex.

2. Total anomalous pulmonary venous connection with obstruction is virtually the only entity that gives congestive heart failure with a small heart.

3. The peripheral arterial desaturation that is consistently present without obstruction may be of such a minor degree as to make the presence of cyanosis difficult to ascertain.

4. In the patient with total anomalous pulmonary venous connection with obstruction, early and prompt diagnosis is essential because the pulmonary edema is life threatening.

5. This is an extremely difficult diagnosis to make, and a high index of suspicion must be maintained when one is looking at any patient who is cyanotic, particularly when the diagnosis is not immediately apparent.

6. A snowman configuration on roentgenogram can be seen in California as well as in Minnesota.

PART IV

Miscellaneous Defects

14

Ebstein's Anomaly

EMBRYOLOGY

At about the fifth week of gestation there is a blending of the anterior endocardial cushion, the posterior endocardial cushion, a portion of the interventricular septum, and the ventricular muscle itself to form the right atrioventricular canal and subsequently the valve, known as the tricuspid valve (Fig 14–1 and 14–2). The papillary muscles and chordae tendineae arise from careful sculpturing of the ventricular muscle (Fig 14–3).

As the leaflets and chordae tendineae develop, so does the conduction system. This specialized muscle with the capability of transmitting impulses passes between the right atrium and the right ventricle. The atrioventricular node is located in the lower portion of the right atrium near the inferior vena cava and the coronary sinus. The bundle of His passes adjacent to the tricuspid valve ring toward the interventricular septum, where it divides into right and left branches, which course along the respective sides of the right and left ventricles.

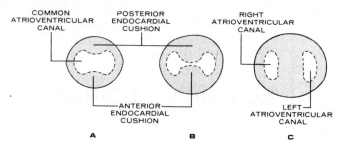

FIG 14–1.

Schematic representation of the common atrioventricular canal developing into a right and a left canal. **A,** 30 days; **B,** 33 days; **C,** 35 days. (See text for explanation.) (Modified from Moss AJ, Adams FH [eds]: *Heart Disease in Infants, Children and Adolescents.* Baltimore, Williams & Wilkins Co, 1968, p 17.)

ANATOMY

If there is disruption of the above mechanism, the tricuspid valve anulus may be displaced downward, incorporating part of the normal right ventricle into the right atrium. The chordae tendineae will be foreshortened, and the total result is this anomaly, in which the right atrium is exceptionally large, the right ventricle particularly small, and the tricuspid valve potentially or actually insufficient (Fig 14–4). Er-

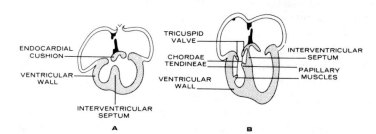

FIG 14–2.

Schematic representation of the formation of the tricuspid valve. (See text for explanation.) Identification of left-sided structures has been omitted intentionally. **A,** 37 days; **B,** newborn. (Modified from Moss AJ, Adams FH [eds]: *Heart Disease in Infants, Children and Adolescents.* Baltimore, Williams & Wilkins Co, 1968, p 16.)

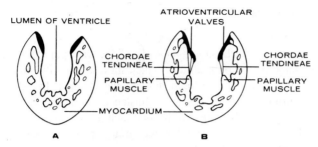

FIG 14–3.
Schematic representation of the formation of the atrioventricular valves and their chordae tendineae and papillary muscles. (See text for explanation.) **A** and **B,** progressive stages of development. (Modified from Moss AJ, Adams FH [eds]: *Heart Disease in Infants, Children and Adolescents.* Baltimore, Williams & Wilkins Co, 1968, p 19.)

rors in developmental patterns can also affect the conduction system. Incomplete disruption of the right-sided bundle can occur, leading to right bundle-branch block. An anomalous pathway across the tricuspid anulus can develop, resulting in the Wolff-Parkinson-White syndrome.

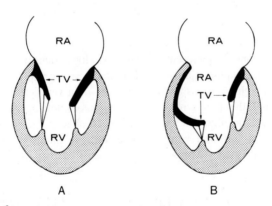

FIG 14–4.
Diagrammatic representation of the anatomical appearance of the tricuspid valve in Ebstein's anomaly. **A,** normal insertion of the tricuspid valve; **B,** displacement of one leaflet of the tricuspid valve. Note the very small right ventricle and very large right atrium. *RA* = right atrium; *TV* = tricuspid valve; *RV* = right ventricle.

HEMODYNAMICS

The patient with Ebstein's anomaly of the tricuspid valve has an exceptionally dilated right atrium, which may secondarily stretch the atrial septum, rendering the foramen ovale incompetent. In the face of tricuspid insufficiency or other circumstances in which right atrial pressure would have increased beyond that of left atrial pressure, right-to-left shunting through the interatrial septum can take place. This concept is depicted in the mnemonic

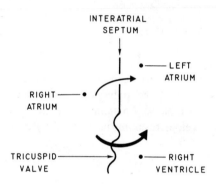

The mnemonic represents a long, patulous tricuspid valve with the interatrial septum above it. The thick arrow represents blood flowing through the tricuspid valve into the right ventricle in a normal fashion, and the thin arrow represents blood flowing through the interatrial septum into the left atrium in an abnormal fashion. If the blood flow is followed with the mnemonic in mind, the effect on the heart and great vessels can be demonstrated by the following diagram:

RIGHT ATRIUM ↑   LEFT ATRIUM →
RIGHT VENTRICLE ↓   LEFT VENTRICLE →
MAIN PULMONARY ARTERY →   AORTA →
PULMONARY VESSELS → ↓

The arrows represent alteration in the size of a chamber or a vessel as follows:

$\rightarrow$ Unchanged
$\uparrow$ Increased
$\downarrow$ Decreased

This information can be translated to the chest roentgenogram, where one would expect to find a very large right atrium, a small right ventricle but with a large outflow tract, which may be confusing, a normal main pulmonary artery, and pulmonary vascular markings that are either normal or decreased (Fig 14–5).

The electrocardiogram (ECG) will show right atrial hypertrophy, absence of right ventricular hypertrophy, and, possibly, left atrial and left ventricular hypertrophy. In addition, and very commonly indeed, will be the presence of conduction defects, such as right bundle-branch block (Fig 14–6) and Wolff-Parkinson-White syndrome (Fig 14–7).

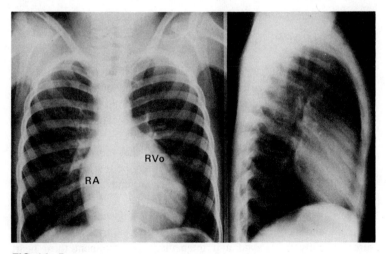

FIG 14–5.
Chest roentgenograms of a child with Ebstein's anomaly. The salient features are a large right atrium and a prominent right ventricular outflow tract. *RA* = right atrium; *RVo* = right ventricular outflow tract.

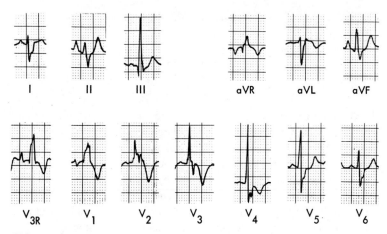

FIG 14–6.
Electrocardiogram of a patient with Ebstein's anomaly showing right bundle-branch block. The salient features are the dominant S₁ and RaVF—right-axis deviation—the wide QRS complex in all leads, and the delayed notched R wave in lead V_{3R} and S wave in lead V_6. Note, however, that the R wave in lead V_1 is not very tall.

CLINICAL APPLICATION

Unless the patient with Ebstein's anomaly of the tricuspid valve is subject to significant tricuspid insufficiency, he or she usually will grow to early childhood with insignificant symptoms. At that time, the patient may have some diminution in exercise capability. Cyanosis may be apparent or so minimal as not to be visible. The patient will appear small to normal in size, with a chest that has a prominent left side. To palpation, the right atrial activity may be felt low in the chest to the right of the sternum, but a classic right ventricular heave should be absent. A left apical thrust may be palpable.

The rhythm of the heart to auscultation is unusual but characteristic. Although the mitral valve closes normally, the tricuspid valve closure generally is delayed and intensified. A prominent third heart sound is common because of filling of the right ventricle. Also, an atrial sound generally is present. This conglomerate of events results in either a triple or a quadruple rhythm. Even though there are two bicuspid valves, the second sound usually is single.

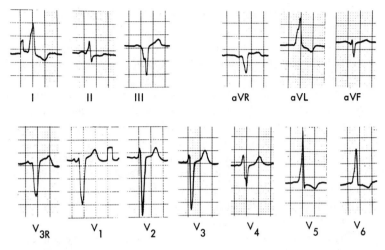

I II III aVR aVL aVF

V$_{3R}$ V$_1$ V$_2$ V$_3$ V$_4$ V$_5$ V$_6$

all ½ standard

FIG 14–7.
Electrocardiogram of a child with Ebstein's anomaly showing the Wolff-Parkinson-White syndrome. The salient features are a short P-R interval in all leads, a very wide QRS complex in all leads, and the slurred initial component of the QRS in most leads—the delta wave.

The most commonly heard murmur is that of tricuspid insufficiency. This early, medium-pitched, rather harsh systolic murmur is heard best at the location of the displaced tricuspid valve and, therefore, would be to the left of the sternum in the vicinity of the fourth or fifth intercostal space.

The cyanosis, when present, is a function of shunting across the atrial septum. Generally, it is only through an unguarded foramen ovale or rarely through a true ostium secundum defect. The quantity of blood flowing through the septum is related to the size of the right atrium and to the degree of tricuspid insufficiency. It should be clear, therefore, why the cyanosis may be minimal to modest. It also should be reasonably clear that the degree of left-sided involvement in terms of left atrial enlargement and left ventricular thrust would be dependent on the size of the intracardiac shunt.

If there is significant tricuspid insufficiency, the patient may get into trouble early in infancy. The diagnosis can be suspected in an in-

fant who is in congestive heart failure with cyanosis, who has a large
right atrium with diminished to normal pulmonary vascular markings
in the chest roentgenogram, and who may have conduction abnormalities in the ECG. A two-dimensional echocardiogram in the apical
four-chamber view can dramatically demonstrate the abnormal relationship of the tricuspid valve (Fig 14–8). This can rather conclu-
sively establish a diagnosis of Ebstein's anomaly. The echocardiogram
will effectively alter the timing of the cardiac catheterization. The latter, rather than serving as a major means of establishing a diagnosis, is
then relegated to the task of defining the effect of the diagnosis at a
time that the clinical course is either unsatisfactory or when surgical
intervention is a consideration. It would demonstrate a large right
atrium with elevated pressures and a small right ventricle with a low
systolic pressure but a high diastolic pressure.

Right-to-left shunting at the level of the atria will be apparent.

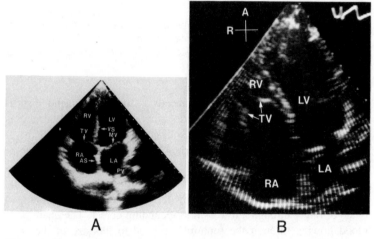

A   **B**

FIG 14–8.
Apical four-chamber view of a normal patient **(A)** and a patient with Ebstein's
anomaly **(B)**. Note in **B** displacement of the tricuspid valve *(TV)* into the cham-
ber of the right ventricle with a resulting very large right atrium. *A* = anterior;
R = right; *RV* = right ventricle; *TV* = tricuspid valve; *RA* = right atrium; *LV* = left
ventricle; *MV* = mitral valve; *LA* = left atrium; *RPV* = right pulmonary vein;
LPV = left pulmonary vein; *MB* = moderator band. (From Silverman NH, Snider
AR: *Two-Dimensional Echocardiography in Congenital Heart Disease.* Norwalk,
Conn, Appleton-Century-Crofts, 1982, p 202. Used by permission.)

The diagnosis can be firmly confirmed with the use of an intracardiac ECG. With the catheter on the atrial side of the tricuspid valve, where there is true ventricular endocardium, a ventricular electrogram will be recorded simultaneously with an atrial pressure curve (Table 14–1).

If the tricuspid insufficiency is negligible, the patient may well grow to early childhood before having either a clinical panorama comparable with that in the infant or merely rhythm disturbances as recognized in the ECG. The diagnosis once more can be confirmed in the catheterization laboratory, as just described.

DIFFERENTIAL DIAGNOSIS

The patient with Ebstein's anomaly must be differentiated from one with congenital tricuspid insufficiency but with normally inserted leaflets, one with pulmonary stenosis and right-to-left shunting through the foramen ovale, and one with Uhl's disease.

TABLE 14–1.

Idealized Cardiac Catheterization Data in a Child With Ebstein's Anomaly*

Site	Pressure (mm Hg) Normal	Pressure (mm Hg) Patient	Oxygen Saturation (%) Normal	Oxygen Saturation (%) Patient
Superior vena cava			70	70
Inferior vena cava			74	74
Right atrium	a = 5 v = 3 m = 4	a = 14 v = 16 m = 14	72	72
Right ventricle	25/2	20/12	72	72
Main pulmonary artery	25/12	20/14	72	72
Pulmonary vein	a = 6 v = 8 m = 7	a = 7 v = 8 m = 8	97	97
Left atrium	a = 5 v = 7 m = 6	a = 6 v = 7 m = 7	97	85
Systemic artery	120/80	120/80	97	85

*The salient features are the elevated pressure in the right atrium and diminished systolic and elevated diastolic pressures in the right ventricle. In addition, the oxygen saturation in the left atrium is decreased when compared with the pulmonary vein. Peripheral saturation is decreased also.

The patient with congenital tricuspid insufficiency characteristically has congestive heart failure at birth. This may be most difficult to differentiate from Ebstein's anomaly, but echocardiography and cardiac catheterization will be of help. With an intracardiac ECG catheter placed near the tricuspid valve, an atrial pressure will be recorded along with a ventricular electrogram.

The patient with severe pulmonary stenosis characteristically has marked right ventricular hypertrophy in the ECG, which should be sufficient to effect a differential diagnosis.

Although the patient with Uhl's disease (underdeveloped right ventricle) does have an effectual right ventricular chamber, it is dilated and has a parchment-thin wall. The tricuspid valve is normal in position, and cardiac catheterization should permit a differential diagnosis.

PEARLS

1. There is no sex preference.
2. The risk of cardiac catheterization is increased because of the high incidence of arrhythmias. However, this should not preclude the study when it is indicated.

15 | Corrected Transposition of the Great Arteries

EMBRYOLOGY

At about the third week of gestation, the primitive cardiac tube begins its earliest changes, which ultimately will transform it into a four-chambered heart. The tube is fixed in its attachments proximally and distally; and growing more rapidly than the pericardial cavity, it folds on itself. The normal folding—called looping—is convex and to the right, which results in the right ventricle being anterior and rightward and the left ventricle posterior and leftward. The atrioventricular valves passively follow their respective ventricles, so the three-leaflet tricuspid valve sits between the right atrium and the right ventricle and the two-leaflet mitral valve between the left atrium and the left ventricle (Fig 15–1). A few days later, the common trunk is divided into two. The caudad spiral growth of the truncoconal ridges results in the origin of the aorta being posterior and leftward, arising from the left ventricle, and the origin of the pulmonary artery being anterior and rightward, arising from the right ventricle (Fig 15–2).

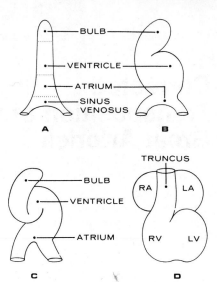

FIG 15–1.
Schematic representation of the development of the primitive cardiac tube into the definitive four-chambered heart. **A,** 18 days; **B,** 21 days; **C,** 23 days; **D,** 28 days. Note the initial rightward convex bending of the tube in **B.** *RA* = right atrium; *LA* = left atrium; *RV* = right ventricle; *LV* = left ventricle.

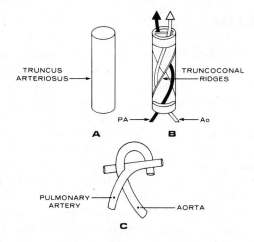

FIG 15–2.
Diagrammatic representation of the division of the truncus arteriosus **(A)** into the aorta and the pulmonary artery **(C). B,** septation and the spiral direction of the pulmonary artery and the aorta are shown. *PA* = pulmonary artery; *Ao* = aorta.

ANATOMY

If, during embryologic growth, the loop does not twist to the right (commonly called *d* loop) but, rather, to the left (commonly called *l* loop), the anatomical right ventricle will be displaced posteriorly and leftward, becoming the arterial ventricle; the anatomical left ventricle will be displaced anteriorly and rightward, becoming the venous ventricle. The common trunk will be septated in a spiral nature but is distorted so that the origin of the pulmonary artery is displaced posteriorly and more rightward, whereas the origin of the aorta is displaced anteriorly and more leftward. Despite the displacement of the great arteries, the pulmonary artery continues to arise from the venous ventricle and the aorta from the arterial ventricle (Figs 15–3 and 15–4).

The right and left branches of the conduction system remain with the appropriate anatomical ventricles. Because the ventricles are reversed in a right-to-left fashion, the position of the conduction system is similarly reversed. In normal circumstances, the interventricular septum depolarizes from the side of the anatomical left ventricle toward the side of the anatomical right ventricle. Since in corrected transposition of the great arteries there is a reversal of the position of the anatomical ventricles as well as the conduction system, and since

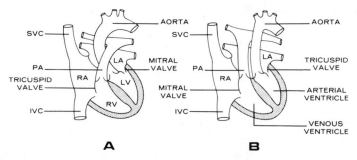

FIG 15–3.
Diagrammatic representation of the anatomical characteristics of corrected transposition of the great arteries. **A,** normal; **B,** corrected transposition of the great arteries. Note that the pulmonary artery arises from the venous ventricle and the aorta from the arterial ventricle. *SVC* = superior vena cava; *IVC* = inferior vena cava; *RA* = right atrium; *RV* = right ventricle; *PA* = pulmonary artery; *LA* = left atrium; *LV* = left ventricle.

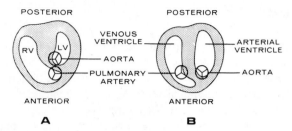

FIG 15–4.
Horizontal sections of hearts showing the great vessel relationship to the ventricles. **A,** normal; **B,** corrected transposition of the great arteries. Note that although in **B** the great vessels are transposed, the pulmonary artery continues to arise from the venous ventricle and the aorta from the arterial ventricle.

the interventricular septum continues to depolarize from the side of the anatomical left ventricle toward the side of the anatomical right ventricle, it should be apparent that, in the patient, the interventricular septum effectively depolarizes from right to left—a reversal of normal. In addition, this abnormal rotation can elongate the bundle of His to such a degree as to result in disruption of its fibers, causing complete heart block.

HEMODYNAMICS

In the absence of any intracardiac defects, the circulation is normal. Venous return is delivered to an anatomical right atrium, from which it passes through a two-leaflet mitral valve into an anatomical left ventricle. It leaves via the pulmonary artery (despite its displacement) into the lungs. Appropriately oxygenated blood returns into an anatomical left atrium, through a three-leaflet tricuspid valve, and into an anatomical right ventricle. It finally leaves via the aorta (despite its displacement) and out the systemic circuit. Therefore, the patient with corrected transposition of the great arteries without intracardiac defects will have a normally functioning heart and may well go unrecognized as having congenital heart disease. However, there are clues to the diagnosis, and these are elaborated on. The basic concept of corrected transposition of the great arteries can be characterized in the mnemonic

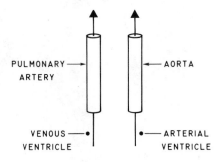

The arrows represent blood flowing from the venous ventricle into the displaced pulmonary artery and from the arterial ventricle into the displaced aorta. If the blood flow is followed with the mnemonic in mind, the effect on the various chambers and vessels of the heart can be demonstrated by the following diagram:

RIGHT ATRIUM →   LEFT ATRIUM →
VENOUS VENTRICLE →   ARTERIAL VENTRICLE →
MAIN PULMONARY ARTERY →   AORTA →
PULMONARY VESSELS →

The arrows represent alteration in the size of a chamber or a vessel as follows:

→ Unchanged

Translated to the chest roentgenogram, one would expect to find a heart normal in overall size but with a peculiar configuration. The aorta dominates the upper left border of the heart, giving rise to an almost straight-line edge to that border (Fig 15–5). Since there is no abnormality in chamber size, the electrocardiogram (ECG) would be expected to be normal. However, because of the abnormalities in the conduction system just noted, it usually is not. Two findings are commonly seen. The first is the presence of a Q wave in leads III, aVF, and V_1 and the absence of a Q wave in leads V_5 and V_6 (Fig 15–6). The second is the presence of complete heart block (Fig 15–7). Despite the logic in this situation, for reasons that are quite unclear, these ECG findings are not seen in all patients.

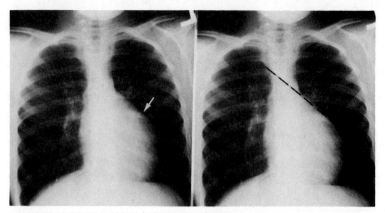

FIG 15–5.
Chest roentgenograms of a child with corrected transposition of the great arteries demonstrating the straight upper left border of the heart representing the ascending aorta (*arrow* in the panel to the *left; dotted line* in the panel to the *right*). (Courtesy of P. Taber, M.D.)

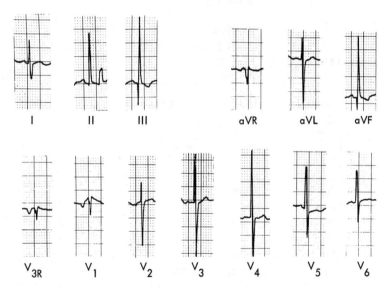

all ½ standard

FIG 15–6.
Electrocardiogram of a patient with corrected transposition of the great arteries, which demonstrates the presence of a Q in III, aVF, and V_1, and the absence of a Q in V_6.

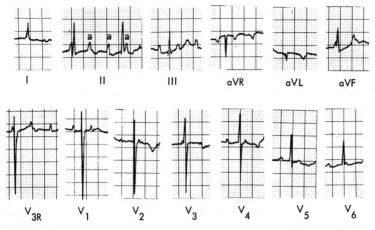

FIG 15–7.
Electrocardiogram of a patient with corrected transposition of the great arteries showing complete heart block. The salient feature is the complete dissociation between the atria and the ventricles. *a* = P waves.

CLINICAL APPLICATION

As has been stated, the patient without a coexisting intracardiac defect can be totally missed and lead a normal life. This is the exception rather than the rule. It is much more common that the patient with corrected transposition of the great arteries has a ventricular septal defect with pulmonary hypertension, an Ebstein-like anomaly of the left atrioventricular valve (the tricuspid valve), pulmonary stenosis, or less commonly, any other intracardiac defect. Since the clinical picture is the result of the intracardiac defect and not of the transposed arteries, a recitation of those findings would be redundant. Therefore, the reader is referred to the appropriate chapters for review, remembering that the basic malposition of the great arteries exists.

DIFFERENTIAL DIAGNOSIS

The patient with corrected transposition of the great arteries and associated defects must be differentiated from one having the same intracardiac defects but with normally positioned great arteries. If complete heart block or the abnormal Q-wave distribution in the ECG or typical chest roentgenographic findings are present, the true diagnosis can be suspected. In the absence of these, however, echocardiography with or without cardiac catheterization will generally be required to establish the diagnosis and define the anatomical details.

PEARLS

1. This defect is more common in males than in females.
2. Coexisting intracardiac defects are the rule rather than the exception.
3. A ventricular septal defect with pulmonary hypertension is the most common lesion seen.
4. This lesion is so complex involving embryology, anatomy, a myriad of coexisting defects, and the abnormality of the conducting system that a clear understanding of it would give an individual deep insight into all of pediatric cardiology.
5. The terms *l*-transposition of the great arteries and corrected transposition of the great arteries are interchangeable.

16 | Hypoplastic Left-Heart Syndrome

EMBRYOLOGY

At about the fifth week of gestation there is a blending of the anterior endocardial cushion, the posterior endocardial cushion, a portion of the interventricular septum, and the ventricular muscle itself to form the left atrioventricular canal and, subsequently, the valve, known as the mitral valve (Figs 16–1 and 16–2). The papillary muscles and

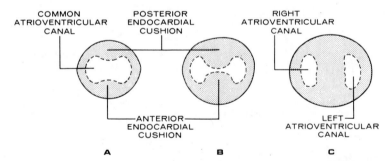

FIG 16–1.
Schematic representation of the common atrioventricular canal developing into a right and a left canal. **A,** 30 days; **B,** 33 days; **C,** 35 days. (See text for explanation.) (Modified from Moss AJ, Adams FH [eds]: *Heart Disease in Infants, Children and Adolescents.* Baltimore, Williams & Wilkins Co, 1968, p 17.)

193

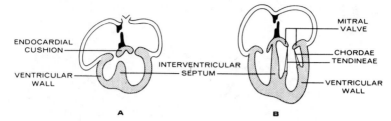

FIG 16–2.
Schematic representation of the formation of the mitral valve. (See text for explanation.) Identification of right-sided structures has been omitted intentionally. **A,** 37 days; **B,** newborn. (Modified from Moss AJ, Adams FH [eds]: *Heart Disease in Infants, Children and Adolescents.* Baltimore, Williams & Wilkins Co, 1968, p 16.)

chordae tendineae arise from the careful sculpturing of the ventricular muscle (Fig 16–3). Slightly later, at about the sixth week of gestation, concomitant with the development of the truncus arteriosus, the aortic valve develops. It is formed by enlargement of three tubercles within the lumen of the aorta, which grow toward the midline and finally are thinned by resorption of excess tissue. There is additional hollowing out of tissue at the superior portion of the tubercle at its junction with the wall of the aorta, giving rise to the sinuses of the valve (Figs 16–4

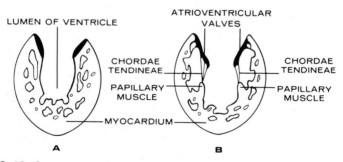

FIG 16–3.
Schematic representation of the formation of the atrioventricular valves and their chordae tendineae and papillary muscles. (See text for explanation.) **A** and **B,** progressive stages of development. (Modified from Moss AJ, Adams FH [eds]: *Heart Disease in Infants, Children and Adolescents.* Baltimore, Williams & Wilkins Co, 1968, p 19.)

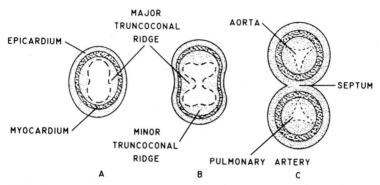

FIG 16-4.
Schematic representation of the formation of the aortic valves within the aorta. Note the progressive proliferation of the truncoconal ridges (the aortic valves are also demonstrated coincidentally). (Modified from Moss AJ, Adams FH [eds]: *Heart Disease in Infants, Children and Adolescents.* Baltimore, Williams & Wilkins Co, 1968, p 16.)

and 16–5). At about the same time, the arches are differentiating, with the fourth arch destined to become the aorta (Fig 16–6).

ANATOMY

If the mitral valve fails to develop totally, mitral atresia will result. If the aortic valve fails to develop totally, aortic atresia will re-

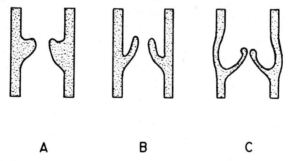

A   **B**   **C**

FIG 16-5.
A graphic demonstration of the proliferation and then hollowing out of the tubercles, giving rise to the completed valve.

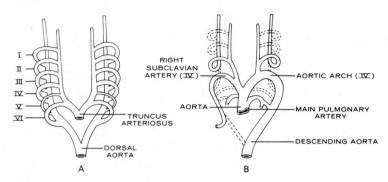

FIG 16–6.
Diagrammatic representation of the embryologic development of the aortic arch system as it relates to the aorta. (See text for explanation.)

sult. If the arch of the aorta does not develop adequately, hypoplasia of the arch will result. Whether because of reduction of inflow due to mitral atresia or reduction of outflow due to aortic atresia or a hypoplastic arch, the common denominator is a diminutive left ventricular chamber (Fig 16–7).

HEMODYNAMICS

It makes little difference whether the aortic valve or the mitral valve is atretic, either individually or in combination, because the dominant burden of both volume and pressure is placed on the right side of the heart. This concept is demonstrated in the mnemonic

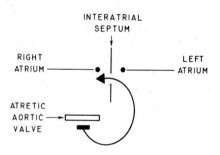

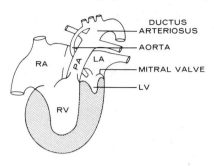

FIG 16-7.
Diagrammatic representation of the anatomical appearance of the heart with hypoplastic left-heart syndrome. Note the diminutive left ventricle, a relatively small mitral valve, and the very small aorta. *RA* = right atrium; *RV* = right ventricle; *PA* = pulmonary artery; *LA* = left atrium; *LV* = left ventricle.

The arrow represents the inability of blood to pass through the aortic valve, with resultant retrograde flow into the left atrium, through the interatrial septum, and into the right atrium. The septum is demonstrated as a line and not a hole to suggest that the passage generally is through the foramen ovale and not through a true atrial septal defect. The same principle would apply if the obstruction were at the mitral valve (this is not demonstrated). If the flow of blood is followed with the mnemonic in mind, the effect on the various chambers and vessels of the heart can be demonstrated by the following diagram:

RIGHT ATRIUM ↑	LEFT ATRIUM ↓
RIGHT VENTRICLE ↑	LEFT VENTRICLE ↓
MAIN PULMONARY ARTERY ↑	AORTA ↓
PULMONARY VESSELS → ↑	

The arrows represent alteration in the size of a chamber or a vessel as follows:

→ Unchanged
↑ Increased
↓ Decreased

Translated to the chest roentgenogram, one would expect to find cardiomegaly with right atrial, right ventricular, and pulmonary artery enlargement. Also, the pulmonary vascularity might be increased.

However, specific chamber enlargement frequently is difficult to recognize in the newborn, and the chest roentgenogram may show only cardiomegaly (Fig 16–8). The electrocardiogram (ECG) would show right atrial and right ventricular hypertrophy with little or no left-sided forces (Fig 16–9).

CLINICAL APPLICATION

The patient with hypoplastic left-heart syndrome is essentially living on blood flow from the right ventricle through the ductus arteriosus into the thoracic and descending aortae. The blood supply to the cerebral vessels and the coronary arteries is merely by retrograde flow. These circumstances place the baby in extreme jeopardy.

The infant may appear to be normal at birth, of average size, and free from either cyanosis or pallor. Shortly thereafter, because of the obligatory intracardiac mixing, these signs will become apparent. The diminished retrograde hypoxemic coronary blood flow ultimately may lead to shock. The peripheral pulses will be small, and the blood pressure, although equal throughout, will be low. The chest will be sym-

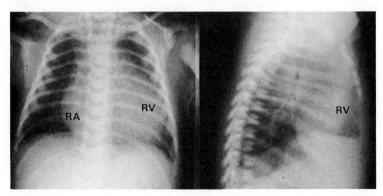

FIG 16–8.
Chest roentgenograms of a newborn with hypoplastic left-heart syndrome. Although there is a suggestion of an enlarged right atrium and right ventricle, the appearance basically is one of cardiomegaly. *RA* = right atrium; *RV* = right ventricle.

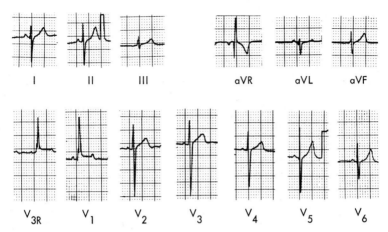

FIG 16–9.

Electrocardiogram of a newborn with hypoplastic left-heart syndrome. The salient feature is the dominant S_I and R/S_{aVF} right axis deviation. Also present are a dominant R wave in V_1 and S wave in $V_{5,6}$, interpretable as right ventricular hypertrophy. The T wave in V_1 is also upright.

metric, and a right ventricular heave will be palpable. The first sound will not be audibly unusual. The second sound will be single, representing closure of only the pulmonary valve (a very important observation). The right ventricle acts as the systemic ventricle. Closure of the pulmonary valve becomes a function of systemic resistance and can be expected to be increased in absolute intensity. Generally, no murmur is heard.

The patient can be suspected of having hypoplastic left-heart syndrome if he or she is believed to be entirely normal at the initial examination and in some 2 to 5 days is found in acute cardiovascular collapse with pallor, poor peripheral pulses, a single second sound, no murmur, and perhaps some cyanosis. This would be the classic presentation. There are, indeed, variations on this clinical pattern where the ventricle can be slightly larger and the picture just described may not occur until 7 to as long as 14 days of age. The presence of cardiomegaly and apparent right-sided enlargement on the chest roentgenogram along with an ECG that shows right ventricular hypertrophy and right atrial hypertrophy will strongly support the clinical impression.

The two-dimensional echocardiogram can exquisitely demonstrate the relationship and size of the ventricular chambers and the nature of both the mitral and the aortic valve. Note in Figure 16–10 that the apex of the heart in a patient with hypoplastic left-heart syndrome is made up by the right ventricle and not the left ventricle when compared with the normal. From this you will hear the term "apex-forming ventricle." Such an observation then will lead to the qualitative and, if necessary, quantitative assessment of the left ventricle size, permitting the diagnosis to be established. If the infant has an umbilical arterial catheter in place, an aortogram can further demonstrate the extremely hypoplastic aortic arch system (Fig 16–11). If further clarification is needed, cardiac catheterization can be employed; it will show an inability to enter or to demonstrate the left ventricle, some left-to-right shunting at the atrial level, systemic pressures in the right ventricle and the main pulmonary artery, normal to low pressures in the systemic artery, and peripheral desaturation (Table 16–1).

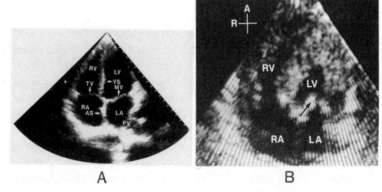

A   B

FIG 16–10.
Apical four-chamber view of an echocardiogram in a normal patient **(A)** and in a patient with hypoplastic left-heart syndrome **(B).** In **B,** note the small left ventricle *(LV)* and *black arrow* pointing to the thickened mitral valve. *A* = anterior; *R* = right; *RV* = right ventricle; *TV* = tricuspid valve; *RA* = right atrium; *LA* = left atrium; *LV* = left ventricle; *RPV* = right pulmonary vein; *LPV* = left pulmonary vein; *MB* = moderator band. (From Silverman NH, Snider AR: *Two-Dimensional Echocardiography in Congenital Heart Disease.* Norwalk, Conn, Appleton-Century-Crofts, 1982, p 191. Used by permission.)

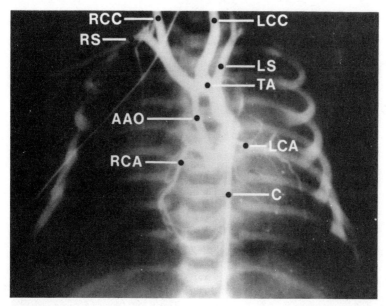

FIG 16–11.
Retrograde aortogram demonstrating very small hypoplastic ascending aorta *(AAO)*. *RCC* = right common carotid; *LCC* = left common carotid; *TA* = transverse arch; *RCA* = right coronary artery; *LCA* = left coronary artery; *C* = catheter; *RS* = right subclavian; *LS* = left subclavian.

DIFFERENTIAL DIAGNOSIS

If the patient with hypoplastic left-heart syndrome is obviously cyanotic, he or she must be differentiated from one having any of the other major lesions causing cyanosis. These are transposition of the great arteries, tricuspid atresia, pulmonary atresia, and, less commonly, truncus arteriosus, total anomalous pulmonary venous drainage, and tetralogy of Fallot.

If the patient is basically pale rather than cyanotic, the differential diagnosis should include consideration of abnormalities of the coronary arteries, such as anomalous origin of the left coronary artery from the pulmonary artery, calcification of the coronary arteries, or, most rarely, thrombosis of a coronary vessel.

TABLE 16–1.

Idealized Cardiac Catheterization Data in a Newborn With Hypoplastic Left-Heart Syndrome*

Site	Pressure (mm Hg)		Oxygen Saturation (%)	
	Normal	Patient	Normal	Patient
Superior vena cava			70	60
Inferior vena cava			74	63
Right atrium	a = 5 v = 3 m = 4	a = 10 v = 8 m = 7	72	78
Right ventricle	60/5	60/5	72	78
Main pulmonary artery	60/40	60/40	72	78
Left atrium	a = 5 v = 7 m = 6	a = 15 v = 10 m = 10	97	97
Left ventricle	60/5	Not entered	97	Not entered
Systemic artery	60/40	60/40	97	78

*The salient features are an inability to enter the left ventricle and elevated pressures in the right ventricle and the pulmonary artery, as well as both atria. Also present are an increase in oxygen saturation in the right atrium and a decrease in the systemic artery.

Interruption of the aortic arch or preductal coarctation of the aorta will also need to be differentiated

PEARLS

1. This anomaly occurs more commonly in males than in females.

2. The echocardiogram is so effective in establishing the diagnosis that cardiac catheterization is only selectively needed.

3. Death within the first week of life is the rule.

4. Splitting of the second sound into two components rules out the diagnosis.

5. The risk of cardiac catheterization in the newborn is 2% to 3% but should not deter one from performing the study when it is indicated.

17

Mitral Valve Prolapse

EMBRYOLOGY

At about the fifth week of gestation there is a blending of the anterior endocardial cushion, the posterior endocardial cushion, a portion of the interventricular septum, and the ventricular muscle itself to form the left atrial ventricular canal and, subsequently, the valve, known as the mitral valve (Figs 17–1 and 17–2). The papillary muscles and chordae tendineae arise from the careful sculpturing of the ventricular muscle (Fig 17–3).

ANATOMY

The mitral valve must be considered as having not only two leaflets, one anterior and one posterior, but also an annulus, chordae tendineae, and papillary muscles. The papillary muscles are firmly attached to the endocardium, which in their own way relate to changes in the myocardium. A malfunction of any part of this apparatus could result in dysfunction of the valve itself.

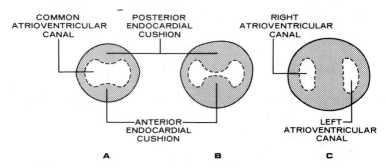

FIG 17–1.
Schematic representation of the common atrioventricular canal developing into a right and left canal. **A,** 30 days; **B,** 33 days; **C,** 35 days. (See text for explanation.) (Modified from Moss AJ, Adams FH [eds]: *Heart Disease in Infants, Children and Adolescents.* Baltimore, Williams & Wilkins Co, 1968, p 17.)

HEMODYNAMICS

Normally the two leaflets are of equal size, open equally during ventricular diastole, and close securely during ventricular systole. During isometric ventricular contraction, there is some billowing of both leaflets into the left atrium, but the orifice of the valve remains securely closed. When the aortic valve opens, ventricular ejection occurs and the left ventricular volume is propelled into the aorta, with none passing the mitral valve.

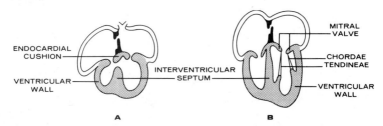

FIG 17–2.
Schematic representation of the formation of the mitral valve. (See text for explanation.) Identification of right-sided structures has been omitted intentionally. **A,** 37 days; **B,** newborn. (Modified from Moss AJ, Adams FH [eds]: *Heart Disease in Infants, Children and Adolescents.* Baltimore, Williams & Wilkins Co, 1968, p 16.)

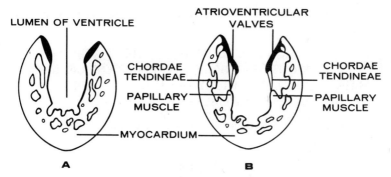

FIG 17-3.
Schematic representation of the formation of the atrioventricular valves and their chordae tendineae and papillary muscles. (See text for explanation.) **A** and **B,** progressive stages of development. (Modified from Moss AJ, Adams FH [eds]: *Heart Disease in Infants, Children and Adolescents.* Baltimore, Williams & Wilkins Co, 1968, p 19.)

In classic mitral valve prolapse, the posterior leaflet of the mitral valve is abnormally large and redundant, as demonstrated in the mnemonic

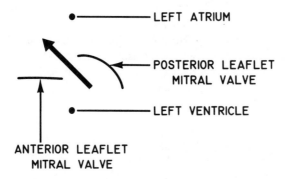

The curved line represents the mitral valve in its prolapsed position, rendering the valve insufficient. The arrow represents blood flow from the left ventricle to the left atrium through the insufficient valve. If the flow of blood is followed with the mnemonic in mind, the effect

on the various chambers of the heart can be demonstrated by the following diagram:

RIGHT ATRIUM →   LEFT ATRIUM → ↑

RIGHT VENTRICLE →   LEFT VENTRICLE →

MAIN PULMONARY ARTERY →   AORTA →

PULMONARY VESSELS →

The arrows represent alterations in the size of a chamber or a vessel as follows:

→ Unchanged

↑ Increased

↓ Decreased

Generally when this lesion is first considered, the degree of insufficiency is negligible, and, therefore, the roentgenogram would be normal. The electrocardiogram (ECG) would have no significant secondary changes and would also be normal. These are not demonstrated. (The role of the ECG and arrhythmias are discussed later in this chapter.)

In mitral valve prolapse, the posterior leaflet of the mitral valve is conceptually abnormally large, and its redundancy is responsible for the abnormal intracardiac hemodynamics. Ventricular diastole is normal. During isometric contraction, the two leaflets of the mitral valve meet each other normally. However, at that point in the middle of systole, eventration of the large redundant posterior leaflet into the left atrium occurs, rendering the valve insufficient. On occasion, the anterior leaflet may also be involved.

CLINICAL APPLICATION

The usual patient is asymptomatic. Somewhere in the patient's life, as early as 3 years of age, but more generally in adolescence or the early teenage years, a murmur, a click, or both at the apex raises a suspicion of mitral valve prolapse. Another common scenario would be the patient's sense of some cardiac irregularity, prompting a visit to the physician. The general examination would be normal. Palpation, percussion, and observation of the chest in such cases is generally not revealing. Auscultation remains the most rewarding exercise.

Keeping the mnemonic in mind, the billowing of the posterior leaflet of the mitral valve into the left atrium in the middle of systole causes a high-pitched sound. This is the click and is identified as a midsystolic, not an early systolic, event. Parenthetically, if the observer believes the first sound to be split, it is much more likely that what is being heard is the normal first sound and a click. This eventration of the valve renders it insufficient and permits a reflux of blood into the left atrium late in systole, which is recognized as the late systolic murmur (Fig 17–4). It may transmit from the apex to the axilla and occasionally may possess an unusual "squeaky" quality, reminiscent of an extracardiac sound. It is of major importance to remember that although the click and the murmur are the hallmarks of the syndrome, their presence may vary considerably with position, certain physiologic or pharmacologic maneuvers, and with time. Events such as standing, presence of tachycardia, performance of a Valsalva maneuver, or the administration of amyl nitrate decrease the volume of the heart shorten isometric contraction and cause the click to move earlier in systole toward the first sound and to make the murmur longer

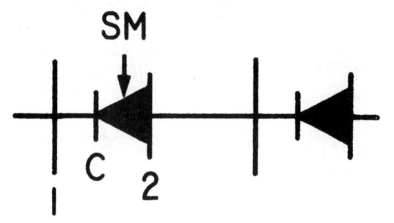

FIG 17–4.
Diagrammatic representation of relationship of midsystolic click and late systolic murmur. *1* = first heart sound; *2* = second heart sound; *C* = click; *SM* = systolic murmur.

REDUCED VOLUME

STANDING
VALSALVA
TACHYCARDIA
AMYL NITRITE

RESTING

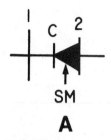

A

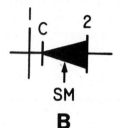

B

FIG 17–5.
Diagrammatic representation of effect of events that reduce cardiac volume on the physical findings of the syndrome. Note movement of click toward first sound and lengthening of systolic murmur. *1* = first sound; *2* = second sound; *C* = click; *SM* = systolic murmur.

INCREASED VOLUME

SQUATTING
BRADYCARDIA
PROPRANOLOL
PRESSORS

RESTING

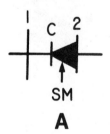

A

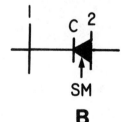

B

FIG 17–6.
Diagrammatic representation of effect of events that increase cardiac volume on physical findings of syndrome. Note movement of click toward second sound and shortening of systolic murmur. *1* = first sound; *2* = second sound; *C* = click; *SM* = systolic murmur.

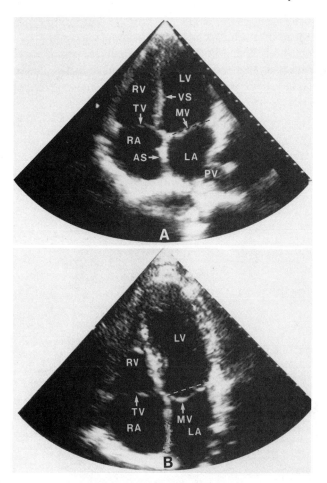

FIG 17–7.
Apical, four-chamber view in a normal patient **(A)** and a patient with mitral valve prolapse **(B).** Note the prolapse of the mitral valve into the left atrium in **B.** The annulus of the mitral valve in both **A** and **B** is identified by the *dotted line. PV =* pulmonary veins; *LA =* left atrium; *LV =* left ventricle; *RV =* right ventricle; *RA =* right atrium; *TV =* tricuspid valve; *MV =* mitral valve; *AS =* atrial septum; *VS =* ventricular septum.

(Fig 17–5). Conversely, events that cause an increase in cardiac volume lengthen isometric contraction, such as squatting, presence of bradycardia, or administration of propranolol or vasopressors, will cause the click to move toward the second sound, making the late systolic murmur shorter (Fig 17–6). These events may be recognized on physical examination.

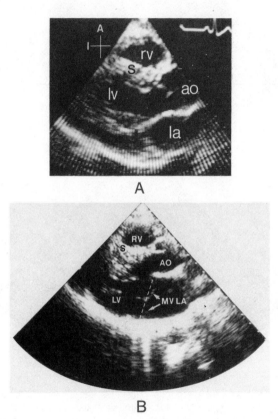

FIG 17–8.
Parasternal long-axis view in a normal patient **(A)** and in a patient with mitral valve prolapse **(B)**. Note in **B** the prolapse of both mitral valve leaflets into the left atrium. The *dotted line* in **B** represents the annulus of the mitral valve. *LA* = left atrium; *LV* = left ventricle; *VS* = ventricular septum; *RV* = right ventricle; *LV* = left ventricle; *AO* = aorta; *MV* = mitral valve.

When the lesion is suspected, a chest roentgenogram and an ECG should be performed even though they will usually be normal. The exception to this is the demonstration, if present, of ventricular or supraventricular arrhythmias. Echocardiography has surfaced as the most widely used laboratory test to confirm the diagnosis. It can demonstrate the abnormal displacement of the posterior leaflet of the mitral valve during midsystole and late systole with a high degree of accuracy in either the apical four-chamber or the parasternal long-axis view of the two-dimensional echocardiogram (Figs 17–7 and 17–8). The

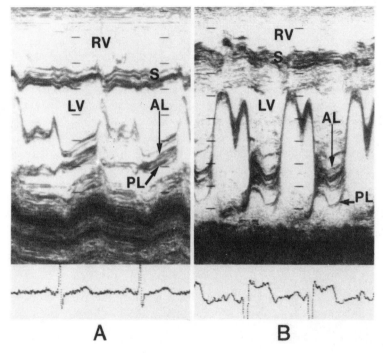

FIG 17–9.
M-mode echocardiogram in a normal patient **(A)** and in a patient with mitral valve prolapse **(B).** Note the late dipping of the posterior leaflet of the mitral valve in **B.** An ECG is seen at the bottom of each panel. *RV* = right ventricle; *S* = septum; *LV* = left ventricle; *AL* = anterior leaflet of the mitral valve; *PL* = posterior leaflet of the mitral valve.

image can be transferred to an M-mode tracing, which can further elucidate the pathology (Fig 17–9). In addition to the classic late systolic dipping, holosystolic dipping beyond an accepted normal level is also interpretable as consistent with the diagnosis.

Although rarely indicated, left ventricular cineangiocardiography performed during cardiac catheterization can further define the syndrome. The redundancy of the abnormal posterior leaflet and, if present, the anterior leaflet can be demonstrated.

The etiology of the syndrome is uncertain. Myxomatous degeneration of the valve is most commonly presented as the cause. Some form of cardiomyopathy has also been implicated. In addition, but perhaps different in pathophysiologic character, is the coexistence of the abnormality with Marfan's syndrome, the straight back syndrome, idiopathic hypertrophic subaortic stenosis, secundum atrial septal defect, and papillary muscle dysfunction secondary to hypoxia of any source. It is also seen in more than one member of the family. For the purpose of this chapter, the lesion has been discussed as an independent entity and not as part of another symptom complex.

A diagnosis of mitral valve prolapse can be suspected in a patient who is either asymptomatic or has cardiac arrhythmias, who has an apical midsystolic click and late systolic murmur. These findings can be evoked by the use of pharmacologic or physiologic events, and the diagnosis can be confirmed with an echocardiogram.

DIFFERENTIAL DIAGNOSIS

Few lesions, if any, mimic this syndrome. The major problem will be in clarifying its existence with or without any other lesion.

PEARLS

1. This is an evolving entity, and one's mind should be open to changes in understanding.
2. Funny "honks" at the apex should raise a suspicion.

3. Overreading of the echocardiogram is common. Be sure of the data before confirming the diagnosis.

4. If arrhythmias are present, a 24-hour Holter recording will assist in the evaluation of the nature of the arrhythmia.

5. The familial incidence of the syndrome is known, and counseling will be of assistance in such instances.

Bibliography

Abrams J: *Essentials of Cardiac Physical Diagnosis.* Philadelphia, Lea & Febiger, 1987.

Adams FH, Emmanouilides GC, Riemenschneider TA: *Moss' Heart Disease in Infants, Children, and Adolescents,* ed 4. Baltimore, Williams & Wilkins, 1989.

Becker AE, Anderson RH: *Pathology of Congenital Heart Disease.* London, Butterworths, 1981.

Elliott LP, Schiebler GL: *X-Ray Diagnosis of Congenital Cardiac Disease,* ed 2. Springfield, Ill, Charles C Thomas Publisher, 1979.

Feigenbaum H: *Echocardiography,* ed 4. Philadelphia, Lea & Febiger, 1987.

Freedom RM, Culhan JAG, Moes CAF: *Angiocardiography of Congenital Heart Disease.* New York, Macmillan Publishing Co, Inc, 1984.

Garson A Jr, Bricker JT, McNamara, D (eds), *The Science and Practice of Pediatric Cardiology,* 3 vols, Philadelphia, Lea & Febiger, 1990.

Gussenhoven EJ, Becker AE: *Congenital Heart Disease: Morphologic and Echocardiographic Correlations.* Edinburgh, Churchill Livingstone Inc, 1983.

Jeresaty RM: *Mitral Valve Prolapse*. New York, Raven Press, 1979.

Keith JD, Rowe R, Vlad P: *Heart Disease in Infancy and Childhood*, ed 3. New York, Macmillan Co, 1978.

Kirklin JW, Karp RB: *The Tetralogy of Fallot: From a Surgical Viewpoint*. Philadelphia, WB Saunders Co, 1970.

Kjellberg SR, Mannheimer E, Rudhe U, et al: *Diagnosis of Congenital Heart Disease*, ed 2. Chicago, Year Book Medical Publishers, 1959.

Long WA: *Fetal and Neonatal Cardiology*. Philadelphia, WB Saunders Co, 1990.

Moller JH: *Essentials of Pediatric Cardiology*, ed 2. Philadelphia, FA Davis Co, 1978.

Nadas AS, Fyler DC: *Nadas' Pediatric Cardiology*. Philadelphia, Hanley & Belfus, 1991.

Perloff JK: *The Clinical Diagnosis of Congenital Heart Disease*, ed 3. Philadelphia, WB Saunders Co, 1987.

Perloff JK: *Physical Examination of the Heart and Circulation*. Philadelphia, WB Saunders Co, 1982.

Ravin A, Craddock LD, Wolf PS, et al: *Auscultation of the Heart*, ed 3. Chicago, Year Book Medical Publishers, 1977.

Roberts WC: *Adult Congenital Heart Disease*. Philadelphia, FA Davis Co, 1987.

Rosenthal A (guest ed): *Pediatric Clinics of North America*, vol 3, no 6. Philadelphia, WB Saunders Co, December, 1984.

Rudolph AM: *Congenital Diseases of the Heart*. Chicago, Year Book Medical Publishers, 1974.

Sacks EJ: *Pediatric Cardiology for the House Officer*. Baltimore, Williams & Wilkins, 1987.

Seward JB, Tajik AJ, Edwards WD, Hagler DJ: *Two-dimensional Echocardiographic Atlas*. New York, Springer-Verlag, 1987, 2 vol.

Silverman NH, Snider AR: *Two-Dimensional Echocardiography in Congenital Heart Disease*. Norwalk, Conn., Appleton-Century-Crofts, 1982.

Snider AR, Serwer GA: *Echocardiography in Pediatric Heart Disease*. Chicago, Year Book Medical Publishers, Inc, 1990.

Taussig HB: *Congenital Malformations of the Heart*, ed 2. Cambridge, Mass. (published for The Commonwealth Fund by Harvard University Press), 1960, 2 vols.

Williams RG, Tucker CR: *Echocardiographic Diagnosis of Congenital Heart Disease*. Boston, Little, Brown & Co, 1977.

Williams RG, Bierman FZ, Sanders SP: *Echocardiographic Diagnosis of Congenital Malformations*. Boston, Little, Brown & Co, 1986.

Zuberbuhler JR: *Clinical Diagnosis in Pediatric Cardiology*. Edinburgh, Churchill Livingstone Inc, 1981.

Index

A

Anatomy
  coarctation of aorta, 85–86, 87
  Ebstein's anomaly, 176–177
  endocardial cushion defect,
    43–44
  hypoplastic left-heart syndrome,
    195–196, 197
  mitral valve prolapse, 203
  patent ductus arteriosus, 31–32
  pulmonary venous connection,
    total anomalous, 158–160
  septal defect
    atrial, 4–5
    ventricular, 14–15
  stenosis
    aortic, 53–54
    pulmonary, 72–73
  tetralogy of Fallot, 109–111
  transposition of great arteries,
    132–133
    corrected, 187–188
  tricuspid atresia, 120–122
  truncus arteriosus, 145–147
Anomalies
  Ebstein's (*see* Ebstein's anomaly)

muscle bundle, and right
  ventricle, 80
pulmonary vein (*see* Pulmonary,
  venous connection, total
  anomalous)
Aorta
  aortic arch system development
    related to, 196
  aortic valve formation in, 55, 195
  coarctation of (*see* Coarctation of
    aorta)
  septation and spiral direction, 108,
    132, 146, 186
  truncus arteriosus division into,
    108, 132, 146, 186
Aortic
  arch
    formation, 86
    system development related to
      aorta, 196
    system development related to
      ductus arteriosus, 32
  insufficiency, echocardiogram, 68
  stenosis (*see* Stenosis, aortic)
  valve
    bicuspid, echocardiogram, 60
    formation in aorta, 55, 195

Aortic *(cont.)*
  proliferation and hollowing out
      of tubercles, 55, 195
  stenosis *(see* Stenosis, aortic,
      valvular)
Aortogram: in hypoplastic left-heart
    syndrome, 201
Arteries
  great *(see* Transposition of great
      arteries)
  pulmonary *(see* Pulmonary, artery)
Atresia *(see* Tricuspid, atresia)
Atrial *(see* Atrium)
Atrioventricular
  canal, common
    developing into right and left
        canal, 121, 176, 193, 204
    division by endocardial
        cushions, 42
  valve formation, 122, 177, 194, 205
Atrium
  interatrial septum formation, 4, 42
  septal defect *(see* Septal defect,
      atrial)
  in shunt *(see* Shunt, left
      ventricular to right atrial)
  sound in pulmonary stenosis, 77

B

Bicuspid aortic valve:
    echocardiogram, 60
Block
  bundle-branch, right, in Ebstein's
      anomaly, electrocardiogram,
      180
  heart, complete, in corrected
      transposition of great arteries,
      191
Bulbar ridges: relation to final fusion
    of ventricular septum, 146
Bulbus cordis: role in
    interventricular septum
    formation, 14, 43, 108
Bundle-branch block: right, in
    Ebstein's anomaly,
    electrocardiogram, 180

C

Catheterization, cardiac
  coarctation of aorta
    postductal, 96
    preductal, 90
  Ebstein's anomaly, 183
  Eisenmenger's complex, 26
  endocardial cushion defect, 49
  hypoplastic left-heart syndrome,
      202
  patent ductus arteriosus, 37
  pulmonary venous connection,
      total anomalous
    above diaphragm, 170
    below diaphragm, 165
  septal defect
    atrial, 9
    ventricular, classic, 20
  stenosis
    aortic, valvular, 63
    pulmonary, valvular, 79
    subaortic, idiopathic
        hypertrophic, 66
  tetralogy of Fallot, 116
  transposition of great arteries, 137
  tricuspid atresia, 127
  truncus arteriosus
    type II, 153
    type IV, 155
Chest roentgenogram *(see*
    Roentgenogram)
Chordae tendineae: formation of,
    122, 177, 194, 205
Cineangiocardiogram
  coarctation of aorta
    postductal, 97
    preductal, 91
  patent ductus arteriosus, 39
  tetralogy of Fallot, 117, 118
  transposition of great arteries, 138
  tricuspid atresia, 128, 129
  truncus arteriosus
    type II, 154
    type IV, 156
Click
  ejection, in pulmonary stenosis, 77

midsystolic, related to late systolic
   murmur, 207
Coarctation of aorta, 85–98
   anatomy, 85–86, 89
   differential diagnosis, 97
   embryology, 85
   pearls, 97–98
   postductal, 91–97
      catheterization, cardiac, 96
      cineangiocardiogram, 97
      clinical application, 93–97
      echocardiogram, 95
      electrocardiogram, 94
      hemodynamics, 91–93
      roentgenogram, 93
   preductal, 86–91
      catheterization, cardiac, 90
      cineangiocardiogram, 91
      clinical application, 88–91
      electrocardiogram, 89
      hemodynamics, 86–88
      roentgenograms, 88
Corrected transposition of great
   arteries (*see* Transposition of
   great arteries, corrected)
Crista supraventricularis: and
   tetralogy of Fallot, 110
Cyanotic heart disease, differential
   diagnosis, 101–106
   guideline to, 102–104
   pearls, 105–106

D

Diagnosis (*see* Differential
   diagnosis)
Differential diagnosis
   coarctation of aorta, 97
   cyanotic heart disease (*see*
      Cyanotic heart disease,
      differential diagnosis)
   Ebstein's anomaly, 183–184
   endocardial cushion defect, 50
   hypoplastic left-heart syndrome,
      201–202
   mitral valve prolapse, 212
   patent ductus arteriosus, 38–40

pulmonary venous connection,
   total anomalous
   with obstruction, 165–166
   without obstruction, 170–171
septal defect
   atrial, ostium primum type,
      10–11
   ventricular, 29–30
stenosis
   aortic, 70
   pulmonary, 83
tetralogy of Fallot, 116–119
transposition of great arteries,
   143–144
   corrected, 191–192
tricuspid atresia, 127–129
truncus arteriosus, 155–157
Ductus arteriosus
   aortic arch system development
      and, 32
   location, and coarctation of aorta,
      87
   patent (*see* Patent ductus
      arteriosus)

E

Ebstein's anomaly, 175–184
   anatomy, 176–177
   bundle-branch block in, right,
      electrocardiogram, 180
   catheterization, cardiac, 183
   clinical application, 180–183
   differential diagnosis, 183–184
   echocardiogram, 182
   embryology, 175–176
   hemodynamics, 178–180
   pearls, 184
   roentgenograms, 179
   tricuspid valve appearance in, 177
   Wolff-Parkinson-White syndrome
      in, electrocardiogram, 181
Echocardiogram
   aortic insufficiency, 68
   bicuspid aortic valve, 60
   coarctation of aorta, postductal,
      95

Echocardiogram *(cont.)*
  Ebstein's anomaly, 182
  endocardial cushion defect, 47, 48
  hypoplastic left-heart syndrome,
    200
  mitral valve prolapse, 209,
    210–211
  patent ductus arteriosus, 36
  pulmonary venous connection,
    total anomalous, with
    obstruction, 164
  septal defect
    atrial, ostium primum type, 11
    atrial, ostium secundum type, 8
    ventricular, membranous, 19
    ventricular, muscular, 21
  stenosis
    aortic, valvular, 60, 61, 62
    pulmonary, valvular, 78
    subaortic, membranous, 68
  tetralogy of Fallot, 115
  transposition of great arteries, 136
  tricuspid atresia, 126
  truncus arteriosus, 152
Eisenmenger's complex, 22–26
  catheterization, cardiac, 26
  clinical application, 24–26
  electrocardiogram, 25
  hemodynamics, 23–24
  roentgenograms, 24
Ejection click: in pulmonary
    stenosis, 77
Electrocardiogram
  coarctation of aorta
    postductal, 94
    preductal, 89
  Ebstein's anomaly
    with bundle-branch block, right,
      180
    with Wolff-Parkinson-White
      syndrome, 181
  Eisenmenger's complex, 25
  endocardial cushion defect, 46
  hypoplastic left-heart syndrome,
    199
  patent ductus arteriosus, 34, 35

pulmonary venous connection,
    total anomalous, with
    obstruction, 163
  septal defect
    atrial, ostium primum type, 10
    atrial, ostium secundum type, 7
    ventricular, classic, 18
  stenosis
    aortic, valvular, 57
    pulmonary, valvular, 75
  tetralogy of Fallot, 113
  transposition of great arteries, 135
    corrected, 190, 191
  tricuspid atresia, 125
  truncus arteriosus
    type II, 149
    type IV, 151
Embryology
  coarctation of aorta, 85
  Ebstein's anomaly, 175–176
  endocardial cushion defect, 41–43
  hypoplastic left-heart syndrome,
    193–195
  mitral valve prolapse, 203
  patent ductus arteriosus, 31, 32
  pulmonary venous connection,
    total anomalous, 158
  pulmonary venous drainage, 159
  septal defect
    atrial, 3–4
    ventricular, 13–14
  stenosis
    aortic, 53
    pulmonary, 71–72
  tetralogy of Fallot, 107–109
  transposition of great arteries,
    131–132
    corrected, 185–186
  tricuspid atresia, 120
  truncus arteriosus, 145
Endocardial cushion(s)
  defect, 41–50
    anatomy, 43–44
    catheterization, cardiac, 49
    clinical application, 47–49
    differential diagnosis, 50

echocardiograms, 47, 48
electrocardiogram, 46
embryology, 41–43
hemodynamics, 44–46
pearls, 50
roentgenograms, 46
dividing common atrioventricular
canal, 42

F

Fallot's tetralogy (*see* Tetralogy of
Fallot)

G

Great arteries (*see* Transposition of
great arteries)
Great vessels: relation to ventricles,
188

H

Heart
block (*see* Block)
catheterization (*see*
Catheterization, cardiac)
development from primitive tube
into four chambers, 186
disease, cyanotic (*see* Cyanotic
heart disease)
left, hypoplastic (*see* Hypoplastic
left-heart syndrome)
sounds in pulmonary stenosis, 77
volume
increase in mitral valve
prolapse, effects of, 208
reduction in mitral valve
prolapse, effects of, 208
Hemodynamics
coarctation of aorta
postductal, 91–93
preductal, 86–88
Ebstein's anomaly, 178–180
Eisenmenger's complex, 23–24
endocardial cushion defect, 44–46

hypoplastic left-heart syndrome,
196–198
mitral valve prolapse, 204–206
patent ductus arteriosus, 32–34
pulmonary venous connection,
total anomalous, with
obstruction, 160–162
septal defect
atrial, 5–7
ventricular, 15–16
ventricular, classic, 16–17
ventricular, small, 20
shunt, left ventricle to right atrial,
26–27
stenosis
aortic, valvular, 54–56
pulmonary, 73–75
subaortic, idiopathic
hypertrophic, 63–64
tetralogy of Fallot, 111–113
transposition of great arteries
corrected, 188–191
with intact ventricular septum,
133–134
with ventricular septal defect,
139–140
with ventricular septal defect
and subpulmonic stenosis,
141–142
tricuspid atresia, 122–124
truncus arteriosus, 147–151
Hypertrophy
in stenosis (*see* Stenosis,
subaortic, idiopathic
hypertrophic)
ventricular
combined, in patent ductus
arteriosus, 35
left, in patent ductus arteriosus,
34
Hypoplastic left-heart syndrome,
193–202
anatomy, 195–196, 197
aortogram, 201
catheterization, cardiac, 202
clinical application, 198–201

Hypoplastic left-heart syndrome
  (cont.)
  differential diagnosis, 201–202
  echocardiogram, 200
  electrocardiogram, 199
  embryology, 193–195
  hemodynamics, 196–198
  pearls, 202
  roentgenograms, 198

I

Interatrial septum: formation of, 4,
  42
Interventricular septum formation
  bulbus cordis role in, 14, 43, 108
  schematic representation of, 14,
    42, 109

M

Midsystolic click: related to late
  systolic murmur, 207
Mitral valve
  formation, 194, 204
  prolapse, 203–213
    anatomy, 203
    clinical application, 206–212
    differential diagnosis, 212
    echocardiograms, 209,
      210–211
    effect of events that increase
      cardiac volume in, 208
    effect of events that reduce
      cardiac volume in, 208
    embryology, 203
    hemodynamics, 204–206
    pearls, 212–213
Murmur: late systolic, related to
  midsystolic click, 207
Muscle
  bundle anomalies, and right
    ventricle, 80
  papillary, formation of, 122, 177,
    194, 205

O

Ostium
  primum defect (*see* Septal defect,
    atrial, ostium primum type)
  secundum defect (*see* Septal
    defect, atrial, ostium
    secundum type)

P

Papillary muscles: formation of,
  122, 177, 194, 205
Patent ductus arteriosus, 31–40
  anatomy, 31–32
  catheterization, cardiac, 37
  cineangiocardiogram, 39
  clinical application, 34–38
  differential diagnosis, 38–40
  echocardiogram, 36
  electrocardiograms, 34, 35
  embryology, 31, 32
  hemodynamics, 32–34
  pearls, 40
  pressure curve in, pullback, 38
  roentgenograms, 33
Pullback pressure curve: in patent
  ductus arteriosus, 38
Pulmonary
  artery
    pulmonary valve formation in, 72
    septation and spiral direction,
      108, 132, 146, 186
    stenosis, peripheral, 81–83
    stenosis, peripheral,
      classification, 82
    truncus arteriosus division into,
      108, 132, 146, 186
  stenosis (*see* Stenosis, pulmonary)
  valve
    formation in pulmonary artery,
      72
    proliferation and hollowing out
      of tubercles, 72
    stenosis (*see* Stenosis,
      pulmonary, valvular)

venous connection, total
anomalous, 158–171
anatomy, 158–160
above diaphragm, cardiac
catheterization in, 170
below diaphragm, cardiac
catheterization in, 165
embryology, 158
with obstruction *(see below)*
without obstruction *(see below)*
pearls, 171
venous connection, total
anomalous, with obstruction,
160–166
clinical application, 162–165
differential diagnosis, 165–166
echocardiogram, 164
electrocardiogram, 163
hemodynamics, 160–162
roentgenograms, 162
vein connection, total anomalous,
without obstruction, 166–171
clinical application, 168–170
differential diagnosis, 170–171
roentgenograms, 168
venous drainage, embryology, 159
Pulse curves: in left ventricular
outflow obstruction, 59

Q

Q wave: in corrected transposition of
great arteries, 190

R

Roentgenogram
coarctation of aorta
postductal, 93
preductal, 88
Ebstein's anomaly, 179
Eisenmenger's complex, 24
endocardial cushion defect, 46
hypoplastic left-heart syndrome,
198
patent ductus arteriosus, 33

pulmonary venous connection,
total anomalous
with obstruction, 162
without obstruction, 168
septal defect
atrial, 6
ventricular, classic, 17
stenosis
aortic, valvular, 57
pulmonary, valvular, 74
subaortic, idiopathic
hypertrophic, 65
tetralogy of Fallot, 112
transposition of great arteries, 135
corrected, 190
tricuspid atresia, 124
truncus arteriosus
type II, 149
type IV, 150

S

Septal defect
atrial, 3–12
anatomy, 4–5
catheterization, cardiac, 9
clinical application, 7–9
embryology, 3–4
hemodynamics, 5–7
ostium primum type, 9–11
ostium primum type,
differential diagnosis, 10–11
ostium primum type,
echocardiogram, 11
ostium primum type,
electrocardiogram, 10
ostium secundum type,
echocardiogram, 8
ostium secundum type,
electrocardiogram, 7
pearls, 11–12
roentgenograms, 6
types, schematic of, 5
ventricular, 13–30
anatomy, 14–15
classic, 16–20

Septal defect *(cont.)*
    classic, cardiac catheterization, 20
    classic, clinical application, 17–20
    classic, electrocardiogram, 18
    classic, hemodynamics, 16–17
    classic, roentgenograms, 17
    differential diagnosis, 29–30
    embryology, 13–14
    hemodynamics, 15–16
    membranous, echocardiogram, 19
    muscular, echocardiogram, 21
    natural history, 28–29
    pearls, 30
    small, 20–22
    small, clinical application, 21–22
    small, hemodynamics, 20
    supracristal, 22
    transposition of great arteries and *(see* Transposition of great arteries, with ventricular septal defect)
Septum
    atrial, defect *(see* Septal defect, atrial)
    interatrial, formation of, 4, 42
    interventricular *(see* Interventricular septum)
    ventricular
        defect *(see* Septal defect, ventricular)
        final fusion and relation to bulbar ridges, 146
Shunt, left ventricle to right atrial, 26–27
    clinical application, 27
    hemodynamics, 26–27
Sounds: in pulmonary stenosis, 77
Stenosis
    aortic, 53–70
        anatomy, 53–54

        differential diagnosis, 70
        embryology, 53
        pearls, 70
        subvalvular, discrete, 67–69
        supravalvular, 69–70
    aortic, valvular, 54–63
        catheterization, cardiac, 63
        clinical application, 56–63
        echocardiograms, 60, 61, 62
        electrocardiogram, 57
        hemodynamics, 54–56
        roentgenograms, 57
    pulmonary, 71–84
        anatomy, 72–73
        clinical application, 75–83
        differential diagnosis, 83
        ejection click in, 77
        embryology, 71–72
        hemodynamics, 73–75
        malignant, 79–80
        pearls, 83–84
        sounds in, 77
    pulmonary artery, peripheral, 81–83
        classification, 82
    pulmonary, valvular
        catheterization, cardiac, 79
        clinical application, 76–79
        echocardiogram, 78
        electrocardiogram, 75
        roentgenograms, 74
    subaortic, idiopathic hypertrophic, 63–67
        catheterization, cardiac, 66
        clinical application, 64–67
        hemodynamics, 63–64
        roentgenogram, 65
    subaortic, membranous, echocardiogram, 68
    subpulmonic *(see* Transposition of great arteries, with ventricular septal defect and subpulmonic stenosis)
Subaortic stenosis *(see* Stenosis, subaortic)

Subpulmonic stenosis (*see*
        Transposition of great
        arteries, with ventricular
        septal defect and
        subpulmonic stenosis)
Supracristal ventricular septal defect,
        22
Systolic murmur: late, related to
        midsystolic click, 207

T

Tetralogy of Fallot, 107–119
    anatomy, 109–111
    catheterization, cardiac, 116
    cineangiocardiogram, 117, 118
    clinical application, 113–116
    crista supraventricularis in, 110
    differential diagnosis, 116–119
    echocardiograms, 115
    electrocardiogram, 113
    embryology, 107–109
    hemodynamics, 111–113
    pearls, 119
    roentgenograms, 112
Total anomalous pulmonary venous
        connection (*see* Pulmonary,
        venous connection, total
        anomalous)
Transposition of great arteries,
        131–144
    anatomy, 132–133
    catheterization, cardiac, 137
    cineangiocardiograms, 138
    corrected, 185–192
        anatomy, 187–188
        clinical application, 191
        differential diagnosis, 191–192
        electrocardiogram, 190, 191
        embryology, 185–186
        hemodynamics, 188–191
        pearls, 192
        roentgenograms, 190
    differential diagnosis, 143–144
    echocardiogram, 136

    electrocardiogram, 135
    embryology, 131–132
    with intact ventricular septum,
        133–138
        clinical application, 134–138
        hemodynamics, 133–134
    pearls, 144
    roentgenograms, 135
    with ventricular septal defect,
        139–141
        clinical application, 140–141
        hemodynamics, 139–140
    with ventricular septal defect and
        subpulmonic stenosis,
        141–143
        clinical application, 142–143
        hemodynamics, 141–142
Tricuspid
    atresia, 120–130
        anatomy, 120–122
        catheterization, cardiac, 127
        cineangiocardiogram, 128, 129
        classification, 123
        clinical application, 124–127
        differential diagnosis, 127–129
        echocardiogram, 126
        electrocardiogram, 125
        embryology, 120
        hemodynamics, 122–124
        pearls, 130
        roentgenograms, 124
    valve
        appearance in Ebstein's
            anomaly, 177
        formation, 121, 176
Truncus arteriosus, 145–157
    anatomy, 145–147
    classification, 147
    clinical application, 151–155
    differential diagnosis, 155–157
    division into aorta and pulmonary
        artery, 108, 132, 146, 186
    echocardiogram, 152
    embryology, 145
    hemodynamics, 147–151

Truncus arteriosus *(cont.)*
  pearls, 157
  type II
    catheterization, cardiac, 153
    cineangiocardiogram, 154
    electrocardiogram, 149
    roentgenograms, 149
  type IV
    catheterization, cardiac, 155
    cineangiocardiogram, 156
    electrocardiogram, 151
    roentgenograms, 150

V

Valve
  aortic *(see* Aortic, valve)
  atrioventricular, formation, 122,
    177, 194, 205
  mitral *(see* Mitral valve)
  pulmonary *(see* Pulmonary, valve)
  tricuspid *(see* Tricuspid)
Vein *(see* Pulmonary, venous)
Ventricle
  atrioventricular *(see*
    Atrioventricular)

hypertrophy *(see* Hypertrophy,
  ventricular)
interventricular septum *(see*
  Interventricular septum)
left
  outflow obstruction, 53–70
  outflow obstruction, pulse
    curves in, 59
  outflow obstruction, types, 56
  in shunt *(see* Shunt, left
    ventricle to right atrial)
relation to great vessels, 188
right
  muscle bundle anomalies and,
    80
  outflow obstruction, 71–84
septum *(see* Septum, ventricular)
Vessels: great, relation to ventricles,
  188

W

Wave: Q, in corrected transposition
  of great arteries, 190
Wolff-Parkinson-White syndrome: in
  Ebstein's anomaly, 181